Insane Euphoria Speaks

Insane Euphoria Speaks

DIARY OF A LATE PREGNANCY

MAY 21, 1971–MARCH 9, 1972

Katherine Dickson

Manguin, Henri Charles (1874-1949) (c) ARS, NY
At the Window, 1904
Location: Private Collection, Avignon, France
Photo Credit: Erich Lessing/ Art Resource, NY

Library of Congress Control Number: 2006907112
ISBN: Softcover   978-1-4257-2801-4

This book was printed in the United States of America.

To order additional copies of this book, contact:
Xlibris Corporation
1-888-795-4274
www.Xlibris.com
Orders@Xlibris.com
32579

Contents

Dedication

To my daughter Jennifer Stephanie

Why discourage women from the colossal swallowing up which is the essence of all motherhood, the mad love (for it is there, the love of a mother for her child), and the madness that maternity represents? For her to feel like a man, free from the consequences of maternity, from the fantastic shackles that it implies? That is probably the reason. But if I answer that men are sick precisely because of this, because they do not have the only opportunity offered a human being to experience a bursting of the ego, how would I be answered? That it was man who made motherhood the monstrous burden it is for sure. But to me the historical reasons for the burden and the drudgery seem the most superficial, because for those there is a remedy. And even if men are responsible for this enslaving form of motherhood, is this enough to condemn maternity itself?

—Marguerite Duras, *Mother to Daughter,*
Daughter to Mother: Mothers on
Mothering—a Daybook and Reader

Friday, May 21, 1971

I decided on Tuesday of this week that I was pregnant. Tuesday night, I told Frank. I expected that he might be unhappy about it. He acted as though he really couldn't conceal his happiness. Sometime ago, I decided that I would like three children. I had had a wonderful pregnancy with Katherine. And after her birth, things were not very difficult although I had anticipated what I had experienced after Thomas, our first child, was born. But nothing like that happened. And I loved Katherine more than anything else in the world, and maybe, that was because the whole experience was not the nightmare that Thomas's birth was. And it seems to me, even to this day, that Katherine is the most beautiful thing I have ever seen. To have another baby now, if I am just given that chance, I could make it a perfect pregnancy. I would really be ready for it, unreservedly ready for it. I could savor everything because it is in a way like sex: it usually takes more than one time to really enjoy it. I think I was happier pregnant with Katherine than I've been at any other time in my life. I was on a permanent high. It helped me recover from Thomas's birth, and nothing breeds success like success, and once I was even a tiny bit happy, it felt so great that I was on an absolute high the whole time. I felt that I was filled with a beautiful surprise, a kind of joyousness in the physical world, a part of nature. It took my pregnancy with Katherine to recover from the experience of Thomas's birth, and yet it seemed that it came almost too soon. It came and was there, and then it was gone; then she was a year old and then fourteen months and sixteen months, and I wanted to hold her. I don't want her to go too fast. I don't want it to be over before I've had a chance to enjoy it. Everything up to this point had been preparation for the enjoyment of this experience. I wasn't ready before. Katherine was a beautiful gift. I mean,

9

having been through what I experienced with Thomas, I just latched on to the happiness I felt with Katherine. It was so welcome. Now, I could really be ready for pregnancy with the full orchestration and the knowledge that it would be my last. This third pregnancy would be just for me. We moved to where we live now only two weeks before Katherine was born, and we went through the whole moving and everything when Thomas was only a year and a half. So it seemed, for such a long time, I was catching up with myself. Now, I think that if I had one more baby, it would just be fun, absolute fun. It would be what Thomas's birth should have been. Some people react to trauma in such a way that they keep going back to the situation, trying to master it. Maybe, that's true for me. I was making up my mind about whether I wanted to have another baby, and then I found out I was pregnant. Maybe, I already knew. I assumed that if I wanted to have another baby, I would have another baby and that I could make that decision. I felt very free about it. And Frank certainly allowed me great freedom, so I felt that it was really up to me, though I sometimes felt that it was gluttonous, and I felt guilty about bringing another child into an already-overpopulated world. I asked Dr. Kuhn if he saw any reason I should not have a third child, and he said no. I told him that in a way, I felt we should perhaps adopt a child if we wanted a third. He said all the homes for unwed mothers are closing down since the advent of the pill, and it's more and more difficult to find children for adoption. I thought that was odd because I had always heard about all the unwanted children, but I guess they are children in other countries that have nobody to care for them. I have since met several women who have said they have not been able to adopt another child. They've called agencies, and there are no babies available now. I don't know whether these are just white children or children that meet other qualifications, but there apparently is a shortage, locally, of babies for adoption.

The one disappointment about Thomas, and also about Katherine, was that I didn't write down any of my experiences about having them; I never really characterized the experience. Also, it seems to me, there is such an enormous gulf in the biological life of a woman—that is, between a woman who has children and is a full-time housewife and the woman who does other things. Even though, now, it is becoming more common for a woman to pursue her career and then take time off for children and then, when the children are very young, to work fewer hours, there is still very little relationship between what she does in her professional life and her children. It seems to me my whole education was completely extrinsic, completely external; it didn't relate to anything at all below the surface. I'm determined to live this pregnancy consciously. I have never read a description by a woman of pregnancy and birth. I think that's absolutely remarkable. One can find things like the *Family of Man* book of photographs, but most of these were taken by men, and these are photographs. I think that the closest thing might be Mary Cassatt's paintings, but then again, they were not her children. She did have a feeling for the relationship between the mother and the child. It seems to me that in so many women who are anxious to have professions and to get an education, there is a bypassing of their biology. They're not really relating their biology to the man's world. I think that what the man's world needs is not just women who will assume the same old roles, but women who really will be different. And I think that there are women who have also experienced women's role, women's experiences, and women's innards—women who know that to be female is to be beautiful.

It's not even six weeks since my last period, but I feel an upward thrust in my uterus, and my breasts feel bigger, and my nipples feel slightly tingly. I feel about three months pregnant. I feel more pregnant than I probably should feel at this point, but it makes me feel very happy. I have something inside, like a beautiful secret that makes me feel very happy. I have a feeling of profound natural happiness.

Wednesday, when we came back home after shopping, I felt so unbelievably tired. Right now, I have a cold, and we came back and both of the children were so fussy and the house was a mess. We had an appointment with the pediatrician, and then we'd gone shopping. I felt I had nothing done. I got home, and I was supposed to call the boy to come and cut the grass but felt I had a thousand little things to do, including filling out Katherine's immunization record, calling a babysitter for Sunday night, calling the Montessori school to make an appointment for Thomas, and getting the library hours from the woman next door. Just then, I happened to look out the window and saw that my neighbor had all her winter clothes hanging on a clothesline to air them. She's got two children, and she works in her house all the time. She cleans her closets and airs her clothes and the draperies. I haven't even gotten my closets organized yet. And I thought of Frank. He probably should buy a new car, and he practically has holes in his shoes, and I thought I must be insane to think about another baby, I mean really insane. It will probably kill us. Now, I can hardly do the work that I have to do. How will I ever manage? I thought maybe the best thing would be not to have the baby, but then I thought, "Well, this probably is my last chance, and if I pass up this chance, it will never happen again, and it will mean more to me as time goes on." I don't want to do this lightly, and I mentioned to Frank that maybe we'd be better-off not to have it. And he said, "Yeah, but then it might be a super kid like Katherine, and then you'd want it." And I think if it were a child like Thomas or Katherine, I would want it so much. I couldn't destroy it. I feel trapped between that and whether or not I can cope with it. I feel like the salmon, driven on by this instinct, but when I finally get to my destination, I'm just going to die.

Thursday, May 27, 1971

It's strange to be married and to talk about the way you really feel because you are torn between saying what seems to you the truth and also not hurting the other person by saying terrible things publicly. I'm sure that if Frank were to read this journal, he would be shocked, but I told him before that I was putting it all down on his tape recorder, and I also told him that he should listen to the tapes, but he hasn't. I do want to get my journal typed and see what it looks like, but I feel guilty about Frank and about paying a typist to transcribe the tapes. What if it's very bad? I don't know. Last Saturday, I felt very guilty because it's like telling tales out of school. Still, in spite of this, there's something that makes me want to do it. Now, I'm waiting for the typist. I've decided to keep this journal on my pregnancy. I would also very much like to write a happy book that comes after the politics of motherhood, either that or it would be an added chapter to what I've done. At the same time, I have an almost-excruciating need for privacy. Katherine and Thomas sleep so little. Some nights, Thomas is up until 11:00 p.m. Frank doesn't get home from work until 9:00 p.m. so we naturally eat at this time as well and by the time Thomas gets in his pajamas and goes through his little nighttime ritual, it's almost eleven. Both children require very little sleep, and there are times, like right now, when I feel exhausted. I feel that I'm in some kind of endurance test. The pregnancy makes me feel exhausted for one thing, and on top of that, I have a horrible head cold. I've had it for about a week. It hurts to read, and my ears ache, and my teeth ache, and my nose and my throat are sore. I feel miserable. There are times when I think I just can't wait for the children to go to bed. It seems that my life would be perfect if I had about one or two hours to myself every day, above and beyond what I have now, which, on many days, is no time at all. I guess all mothers of young children feel this way, but I have been wondering what I should do about this pregnancy.

I went to Dr. Kuhn's office yesterday and had a pregnancy test, and it's positive. It's been six weeks since my last period, and I just wonder whether to have the baby or not. I keep trying to figure out what I really want to do, and the trouble is that before I got pregnant, I couldn't make the decision about whether or not to have another baby, and part of it was that if ever Frank said, "No, I don't think we should," that would make me feel I want to because nobody was going to say that I couldn't do such and such. Now that I am pregnant, I'm sure that my thinking is colored by my feeling exhausted and having this cold. Taking care of Katherine and Thomas is all the more difficult, and I wonder whether I can survive. Frank has done nothing downstairs on the basement, and there are so many factors, but one thing I must say is I feel that it's up to me. I mean, it's really up to me.

It really is a beautiful thing to have a baby, or it should be, and I feel that it's only now that I'm ready for the experience. I don't think I got out of my pregnancies with Katherine and Thomas all that I could have. I should have really learned much more from them. It would have extended that mother period of my life a little longer. Otherwise, it would be completely over. Katherine will be two in September. I hate to see that period end. It's like people who look at their children and say, "Where did their childhood go? I never really enjoyed them." I don't want that to happen to me. On the other hand, it just seems that Frank and I move so slowly it would overwhelm me to have another child. I think it would just about kill me. Maybe, if I got over my cold, I would feel better about it. Crying in the night and getting up in the night, and Katherine at the stage she is, neither in her high chair nor out of her high chair. When she's up, I cannot take my eyes off her for a minute. We cannot afford another baby. Frank needs a new car.

I had a card from Connie, a beautiful card with a blue background and a green flower on it, which was designed by Winnie. Connie said that she went to a program at the MIT Center for Advanced Visual Studies, and she heard Gyorgy Kepes speak. She said that he really was great, and I thought, "How I loved that job in the MIT Rotch Library, with Kepes there and the faculty doing exciting things now," and I was thinking it would have been better if I hadn't left there. I do think that sometimes, but in a way, I had to leave; otherwise, I never would have been able to cut the umbilical cord of formative influences. If I could have gone to a Kepes lecture once a week, I think I could have lived off this and been sustained by it. I think I never would have really done anything myself. There would always have been something stimulating going on, cultural events and other exciting things, and then there would always have been somebody that I knew that was going to whatever the event was and it would have been great to talk to that somebody about it afterward. I would have been forever eating meals that other people had cooked and never be doing my own. Leaving put me alone in my own desert, going down, as George Nakashima, the furniture maker, said, into the headwaters and leaving civilization to find some little space to crawl into and begin to create cells. I never would have taken the time to do that. I don't know whether I will be able to create anything here. In a way, you could say I've created two fantastic children, so from that point of view, I'm glad that I had a chance to leave because I do think that Anna was right when she said a long time ago, when Frank and I were going to get married, that if I stayed there very much longer, I wouldn't be able to leave. I can imagine the kind of ideal life that I would have had if I'd continued working there and been married and had my two children. But maybe, I would not have grown the way I think I would have hoped to grow. Life in Boston didn't take everything, but I did give a great deal, and I don't think that I would have been able to live that life and this life too. I probably would have hired somebody to take care of the children.

What I want to do is create a life, create as much beauty as Kepes. Maybe, I had to come here to do it. What I would really like to do is unite the two halves of a woman. I've got to start creating my own beauty and stop living off Frank and other people. The card from Connie was interesting because it was handmade by a friend.

Last Sunday, we had an episode with roaches. Frank put roach powder around and used roach spray. Frank was ugly, disagreeable, in a bad mood, as though he's terribly put-upon and deprived. Everything I said he disagreed with. Maybe, it was because of me putting an ad in the paper for the typist. He told me, "Yes, go ahead if you want to." Maybe, it was because of the pregnancy. He acts as though he thinks I'm a not-good-enough housekeeper, and maybe, that's because I have been doing this recording. Thomas was three in March, and it was about that time that I started this recording. For three years, I had done nothing in the way of reading or recording or any of the things that I have wanted to do, and Frank always told me in a very abstract way, "Do your own thing. Do what you want to do." But his standards are so inconsistent. In the morning, he likes to sleep, and I feel bad if I even run the vacuum cleaner or the dishwasher. Then when he gets up, if I ask him to watch Katherine while I run down to put things in the washer, he gets up and acts as though he wants to tell me all his fantasies. If I'm busy trying to watch Katherine, cook, and clean, I feel as though it's insulting to him. Yet if something isn't right where he thinks it should be or something comes up like the roaches, he acts like a martyr.

He got mad with me for going to Dr. Kuhn's on Wednesday. I had wanted to have the pregnancy test so badly, and I mentioned it to him, and he said, "No, no, don't have it. What's the point in having it? Have it later." I wanted to have it right away so if I did decide that I wanted an abortion, I at least would have enough time to make a decision. Every time I mentioned it, he said, "You don't know." Finally, Tuesday night, I said, "I'd like to go to Dr. Kuhn tomorrow." And he said, "Thought we were going to get Thomas shoes?" And I said, "We can still get his shoes, and I'll help you downstairs with the nails." Wednesday morning, I said, "Do you mind if I go down to Dr. Kuhn's?" And he said, "Well, yeah, I do." That was inconsiderate of him to take that attitude, I thought. I had to cajole him a bit so that I could go.

Yesterday, he was in a most unbearable mood. When I came back from the doctor's and had finally got the kids in for their naps, he came into the living room and sat on the sofa, trying to fix the can opener. He acted like a mad man. He kept swearing at the can opener. I couldn't talk to him. I couldn't get over the fact that the phone's ringing bothered him so much. The first few times that this happened, I felt fantastically guilty. I would feel as though I had done something wrong. It always turned out that it was a very important reason this person called. One day, my sister, Louise, called. I thought that the call was semiurgent. Frank kept saying, "It's started to rain. You better go and get Thomas." And I said, "Well, Frank, why don't you go out and get him? I'm on a long-distance phone call. I'm only going to talk about five more minutes at the most. You go out and get him." There were so many abrasions. When he comes in from work, I can see that it is an imposition, I understand that, and I never make calls at that time. Only once has it happened, and again, it was a call from my sister. People probably think that our hours are more conventional and that Frank gets home early in the evening and eats earlier. What strikes me about these incidents is that I feel guilty the way I did the night I was talking to Louise on the phone. I think it was about eight-thirty at night. I did talk to her only a few minutes longer, and then I hung up. He said to me, "Kids kill themselves. Don't you care? You can phone anytime." When these incidents occur, there is always a tinge of guilt; it's a hangover from an era when a husband had control of all of his wife's time. What prison is this? Then there would be a fight. When Frank acts that way, it seems as though it's because of me that he's acting that way; it reflects the way he sees me. I want him to think that I'm just great, and when he acts dissatisfied with me, it makes me feel dissatisfied with myself, and I make excuses. I didn't have time, or I did the best I could, or I've been sick all week. It makes it worse. I temporarily see myself by his standards, and I end up hating myself. Whether it's because of the disagreeable things we've said or because I agree with his low opinion of me, I feel terrible, and I feel the need to be purified.

Monday, it took me hours to get myself back to a feeling of grace. I decided that deep down, I am happy, and I don't want my image of myself to be distorted by the way Frank acts. I must be brave enough to be myself. In a way, I think I see through some of these things and see why they bother me the way they do. Still, it hurts me that Frank seems so dissatisfied with me.

Sunday, May 30, 1971

After the roaches, I felt I wanted to take a shower to get rid of all these bad feelings. Monday, it took me hours to get myself back to a better frame of mind. Deep down, I am happy, and I don't want my image of myself to be distorted by what Frank says or does. I want to be me, and I want to be brave enough to be myself. In a way, I think I see through some of these things and see why they bother me the way they do. It seems that Frank is dissatisfied with me, and yet if I call it to his attention, he says no. Yesterday, when he went out, he had said something, and I said, "What?" He seemed to be so mean to me. I asked him if he wanted some coffee, I said, "I'll pour some coffee." He said, "Well, I can't stop for it now." And then he sat with the children, and we were supposed to be having a conversation with them. Today, he asked me if there was anything that he could pick up from the drugstore because he knows that I have this awful cold. "You could get me some oranges and a candy bar." He said, "You shouldn't be having any candy bars if you're pregnant." He sets the things up so that he can refuse me. Then he said, "It seems that with everything I say, you say 'what'." I almost said, "What?" But I didn't. These things are not going to upset me so much anymore. I feel more and more that I'm coming into my own. I feel that this baby is entirely up to me, and I'm not going to be the repository for Frank's bad feelings. He's so unconscious of the way he's operating, these contradictory whims. He goes by his own inner clock. When it's his time to get after the roaches, it's time to get after the roaches, and everybody else should also get after the roaches. And when it's time for him to stay in bed and read, it's time for him to stay in bed and read, and if somebody else needs to work on insect problems, well, that's just too bad. He's not aware of this. I can say that I think I don't let these things bother me anymore. I feel that there are more reasons for me to be here on earth than paddling behind Frank. I don't know. Part of the reason that I do feel the way I do is not just because of the way that he treats me, but the way he responds when I mention it to him. "Well," he says, "how do I treat you?" I never know what to say. It is an impasse. I have been reading David Cooper's *The Death of the Family*, and he says more or less that when two people get married, it's a mutual suicide pact and that one becomes the other's parasite. You look inside a person and what do you find? You find his mate.

I keep thinking about this baby and what to do about it. During most of my pregnancy with Katherine, except for the first two months when I felt miserable, I felt ecstatic all the time. I felt that I loved Frank so much. I think he really outdid himself trying to do things for me. I wish that I were really great, but it's so hard when I don't feel well and the kids can grind me down to a nub. I feel subhuman sometimes. I'm beginning to come into my own. I know that I'd like to keep this journal, and then I'd like to do either a happy book or else do the happy book as a last chapter to the motherhood work and the other things that I'm writing about. When I have some time to myself, life is so great, so fabulous, and wonderful, like right now. I adore looking out at the leaves. Everybody needs a little time for themselves and a little privacy, but there are just so many things to do.

When I think about an abortion, I feel that I'd like to get all the facts so when I decide to have the baby, I can say that I really decided to have it. I called Columbia Hospital for Women. They perform abortions on women who are District of Columbia residents, and they perform them up to twelve weeks. This is covered by Blue Cross and Blue Shield Association. The person that I talked to led me to believe that private doctors in the district can do them for an outside-the-district resident. Tomorrow morning, I will call Kuhn's office and see what his nurse says. I would guess that, probably, Dr. Kuhn's office would refer patients to some other doctor who would then perform them in Columbia Hospital. Perhaps, the Dr. Waters who sells diaphragms. Dr. Kuhn's a Roman Catholic and won't do it. Everything is up to me. I want to eliminate the distance between subject and object, between the objective world and the subjective world. I think that's one thing that I can do through these tape recordings, give some kind of shape to the way I feel and think in the form of a personal journal.

I was talking to Roselle and Shirley. Both of them are pregnant, and both are expecting babies in November. Roselle says that she always wanted to get married and have children, and she really wishes that she could stay at home. I asked her what she thought of Women's Liberation, and she said, "Oh, not much." She thought that equal pay for equal work was okay, but that's all, and she's doing her thesis on married women graduate students at Howard University. She's finishing work on her masters, and she's expecting her second baby. She is twenty-eight years old. She wanted to become a Montessori teacher, but the training program she'd have to go through is too long. She probably will stay at the library. She's admirable really, working and going to school and having children. But it isn't what she wants. She wants a kind of suburban life. I think she thinks that my life is ideal. I don't think she's interested in what she is taking up at school. It isn't something close to her heart. I think she's just doing it because with a master's degree, she'll probably get a grade 11. She could probably have that project and make good money. But the job isn't a career to her. It's just a job. She's so accomplished but so uninvolved. These things are all forms that she goes through. She doesn't really give anything. She was a debutante.

When she was growing up, because she was the minister's daughter, she always felt that she had to be perfect; all eyes were on her, and she couldn't really do what she wanted to do. And you know, her whole life is like that in a way. It's a shame that she's not doing something that she wants to do, that she cares about. I was very glad that Shirley is expecting a baby. But is it possible to be married and have babies and go to school and be involved in something that you really want to be involved in all at the same time? It gets easier all the time, I guess. It's amazing to me now that I'm pregnant for the third time that this is the first time I've thought it would be quite easy. Certainly, it's legal to have an abortion, but I think that it would be harder for Roselle to do all these things if she were also doing something that she really loved and her husband were also doing something that he loved, but I think her husband is not doing very much of anything.

This morning, we had an appointment at the Montessori school. We sat in on classroom activities there. It's amazing! All the things there are kid size. The children were about five years old, and they were sitting down at little tables with scissors, all doing different things. The little girls on the floor were playing with a big dishpan with soapsuds in it. I was very impressed by the teachers. They looked just great. They looked like Jane Smith. Kettering Elementary may be just great. They may have a super kindergarten over there. I don't know. But the teachers at the Montessori school are down on the floor with the kids, and the kids are encouraged to interact with their environment. It's great. I was sitting there thinking about this thing I read. It was the *Equals One*, the magazine that Anna sent me about a year ago. It was about a book by George Leonard called *Education and Ecstasy*. The function of most education is to just keep the new generation from changing things too much, to further the status quo. Education and ecstasy should be about the same. It's not just the learning of a bunch of things but enlightenment: an experience that really changes you—you should really be transformed by it and not just indoctrinated or propagandized. While I was sitting there, I was thinking I wish I could do more with my children, I wish I didn't have housework or cooking to do, and I wish I could play with them all the time and sleep when they sleep. That would be so great! That's what would be great about having another baby: it would be a fulfillment of this possibility. I'm still trying to decide what to do. When I went over to the Prince George's Community College Library, I got out Eleanor Bertine's collection of essays called *Jung's Contribution to Our Time*. Bertine says that any human experience may be a maze in which to wander to destruction or a laboratory for the creation of consciousness depending on the way it is met. And I think that in the tapes that I did before, the motherhood tapes, that was one thing that struck me about my relationship with Frank: you can almost make it heaven or hell. I felt, after a while, as though I could destroy him if I wanted to. I have to work toward not destroying him and not letting him destroy me. Just as with this baby, it seems that you can give birth to it or destroy it, and it's true that the mother has so much power in her hands for either the good or bad of the children. I guess that's why Cooper could write his book. People who are good to you, your friends or your mother, are also the only real enemies that you ever have in any kind of ordinary life experience situation, unless you get machine-gunned, for instance. People are conscious only to such a small extent, and they have such capacities to go either way.

Tuesday, June 2, 1971

Frank has been home from the office over the long Memorial Day weekend, and Frank and his father did some work downstairs during that time. I still have my horrible cold. It's one of the most uncomfortable colds I've ever had, mostly because it has dragged on and on. Yesterday was the worst it has been. I think it is better today. It has rained and rained and rained. The combination of the cold and the rain is too much for me. At least, I don't feel as though I have to take the children out; it is easier to mind them indoors, at least Katherine is. But Thomas did go out for a little while with his boots and his slicker.

The past few days, I have felt exhausted, and it's more than exhaustion; I feel overwhelmed. I want to stand absolutely still and feel cosmic vibrations or something that can generate some energy in me. I want to stand open-mouthed and gulp in some energy. I'm sure that this is the pregnancy. Just to breathe deeply would be enough. I am so far behind on the little things, just haven't gotten them done, though, in a way, it's amazing that I've done as much as I have.

Friday, I got Thomas to playschool and then to the dentist for his appointment in the afternoon, and Thursday morning, we went to the Montessori school, but all the time, I have been wondering, still, whether to have the baby or not. It's completely in my hands, and I've been thinking about it, and my thinking has been colored to some extent by the way I feel. I mean I feel so psychologically overwhelmed that I wonder if I will be able to cope. Maybe, it's just crazy for us to go through with it because we need so many other things and the amount of effort that goes into the baby, at least for me, is enormous. I wonder if the women who know me

21

would think that it's too much, that I would be spreading myself too thinly. It's not that I'm bound by what other people think, but I do wonder if I can manage to do all there is to do. When I think of all those diapers and getting baby clothes ready, I don't know. Feeling the way I've been feeling hasn't helped. I wonder if my body is producing estrogen and if that's the reason I feel like a blank; there's a big blank feeling all around me, and maybe a lack of hormones, the lack of estrogen is causing it. Feeling that and this feeling of being overwhelmed coming at the same moment are very peculiar. It's as though, as far as the eye can see, there is nothing but chores, and life just seems blank. I should be in bed, and yet I'm up trying to do things.

Saturday afternoon, it rained and rained and rained, and Katherine woke up from her nap at about 2:00 p.m., and I decided that I would try and change the sheets on our bed and vacuum and dust our bedroom. Partly because I was looking out to check on Thomas and because Katherine Louise was with me, it took me about two hours to do that; lifting the corners of the mattress to tuck in the sheet seemed like lifting the heaviest thing. I felt as though I were coming to a complete halt, going into a blank. My thoughts aren't even interesting. There seems to be nothing to look forward to; there is only this blank.

Last night, I was cooking dinner for all of us and for Frank's father, and I was cooking steak and some frozen vegetables, and I decided to do it during the time that *Sesame Street* was on so that Thomas would be busy watching the show. Well, the whole time that I was trying to cook, poor little Katherine Louise wanted my attention, and she was pulling at my legs, and she was trying to play tunnel between my legs. She would bump her head on the cabinet under the sink, and I would pick her up and hold her for a couple of minutes and try to distract her a little bit and put her down again, and she would start to cry. It was so difficult to try to cook a meal while she was fussing. It's hard enough just to listen to the fussing, but to try to get a meal done at the same time wears me down. Then she would come into the living room and Thomas would hit her. The kitchen and the living room were covered with the kids' toys. It was hot; I felt horrible. Then I looked at our neighbors next door who were sitting outside, drinking cans of beer before their cookout, and they had five kids over there running around, playing, not requiring the slightest bit of attention. No sooner did we sit down to eat than Katherine dumped over her orange juice and threw the cup on the table. She wants her dinner faster than I can cut up the meat, and then when I give it to her, she's finished eating it in about a second. She doesn't like what's on her plate; she's ready to give back the plate before I've started eating. She's standing up in her high chair, and her hands need to be wiped off. I started to get her ready for bed. I put her into bed about three times before she finally went to sleep. She'd drink a little of her bottle and then start to cry and stand up. Then out the window, I was watching Thomas and these same people next door who were having a barbeque. Thomas was a couple of feet from their table, lying on the grass, watching them. I felt bad that they didn't offer him anything to eat. But afterward, I felt there's no reason they should, and probably, they would actually check with me first. Then I thought of all the times I could have given Thomas some attention, and I didn't. Why should I feel bad about a neighbor not giving him something? I wondered if I've given him something of myself every time I could have.

Between getting Katherine up out of bed and putting her back into bed, I felt so hot and uncomfortable. I was beginning to go blank again. Then I couldn't see Thomas anymore, so I decided to call Rina Plow and see if he was there, but Katherine was making so much noise I couldn't even hear Rina, except that she was saying, "Do you want him to come home?" and I was saying, "Would you tell him that I want him to come home." I looked out the window and saw Rina come out of her house, smoking a cigarette, looking around for Thomas, and I felt horrible because she was probably sitting down having a cigarette, and I called and she had to get up and look around for Thomas. I felt like an idiot.

Eventually, Thomas came home, but Katherine was still up, and I was trying to give Thomas a bath. I did finally get him into the tub, but he didn't want to get washed, and it seemed as though he was so balky, so grouchy, so negative, and uncooperative. Then he doesn't want those pajamas—he wants some other pajamas—and he wanted his shirt under his pajamas, and then he wanted his shirt over his pajamas, and it was 10:00 p.m., and I had just gotten Katherine to sleep. Thomas had not had a nap for three days, and he was out playing and running around rain or shine, so I knew he was exhausted. It wasn't that I was putting him into bed because I just wanted him to go to bed. After the pajamas and shirt were resolved, he wanted milk, and then he wanted juice. It took him about two hours to drink each one of these glasses. It was excruciating. Finally, I guess it must have been about 11:15 p.m. when I finally put him into bed and sat down. I was in a state of collapse. I wanted to get up and have a cup of tea, but I didn't feel I had the strength to do it, and Frank wanted me to go downstairs and look at the paneling he had put up.

Do I want to have another baby? I had felt earlier that all I do is just put stuff away. The number of things that I put away is uncountable, and still, it seems there is a lot of clutter everywhere and still more stuff that I need to put away: all the dirty clothes and all the clean clothes and the dishes. It takes hours every day just to keep those counters somewhat cleared off, not completely cleared off. I feel too tired even to have thoughts.

Yesterday morning, I don't know how I managed to do it, but before Frank's father came, I picked up all the toys from the living room rug, vacuumed the rug, put away a dishwasher load of clean dishes, put the dirty breakfast dishes into the washer, cleared off the counters, and cleaned up all the crumbs and drips and drops. I had managed to put clothes in the washer and had given Katherine a bath. I don't know how I managed to get all the things done. The house did look reasonably neat, but I seemed a joyless blank in it. This is all an oppressive round of chores. If I don't either feel better or do these chores, I'll be communicating to the children such a lack of joy, a lack of life's joy. Their mother is a completely hard-pressed person. I am like Mrs. Rip Van Winkle, not with her sharp tongue, but with her never-smiling, martyred face. And I thought, "Well, I can let these feelings destroy me if I want to. My enemy is this streak in me that makes me do these chores, and I end up unsmiling."

Last night, I felt it was impossible for me to smile. I don't want the children to have that impression of me. I want the impression to be a feeling of liberation, real joy, and fun. Yesterday morning, I was up with the kids at seven-thirty. Frank got up just about the time that his father came, about eleven. Frank had some coffee. I feel jealous when he's in bed and sleeps about three hours more than I do in the morning, and I'm the one that's sick. Then when he gets up and is reading a magazine, I say to myself, "Well, I can sit down and read a magazine too; a certain chore won't get done, but after all, that is my choice, and I can make a choice between the two and live with the fact that the chore isn't done."

One thing I must say about Frank is that he may not accomplish anything, but he does things in his own time, and there is nothing that I can do to change him. He does seem to enjoy life in his own way, at his own pace. He has a lot of fun with the children, and he manages to find time to relax and do things. When his father came over, Frank was in his pajamas, and his father kept saying, "Come on, come on, let's get started. Let's get this job over with," and Frank's father said to me at one point, "You know, Frank is a staller." It was funny because Frank's father was saying, "Last night, I was up all night worrying about this job, and I was worrying about that wiring." It was funny because Frank was supposed to be checking a book on wiring, and instead, Frank is reading *Time* magazine. Here, it's Frank's basement, and his father is the one who's doing all the worrying about it. When his father comes, Frank whips out his wiring magazine and is looking the thing up. It's a riot, but it's a credit, I guess, to Frank's intelligence that he does as well as he does. Instead of wanting to get some chore out of the way so that the rest of the time he'll have for himself, it's just the opposite with him. I think that he feels that if he starts to do a chore, it's likely to just stretch out forever. So the best thing to do is just relax until five minutes before the thing has to be done and then, somehow, worry about it then. If Frank needs directions for going someplace, he never looks up the directions ahead of time. He always waits until he's going there. He'll stay lost forever. Eventually, he'll find it; he always does.

The big lesson that the kids have taught me is to enjoy life and delight in it and save a few minutes for the chores. If they get done, they get done. If anything is pressing enough, somehow, it gets done. But yesterday, I thought, "I can destroy myself with these feelings." And yesterday, while Thomas was out and I was trying to get Katherine to bed, Freddy Plow came up and got on the tyke bike. I went out after him. I said, "Freddy, don't ride that bike," and he went right on riding it. He completely disobeyed me. Watching Thomas out the window and hoping that the kids won't hit him, that he plays well, and then this whole business about the kids' toys, it drives me wild. Do I want another child and have to go through all this all over again? I just couldn't save myself from my own feelings of being driven by all these chores and from feeling sorry for myself. I am sick, and I'm not in bed.

The other night, my mother called, and I know she called because she hadn't heard from me because I was supposed to send a photo back to her and I'm just sending it back now. My mother sounded sad. Ever since my sister, Louise, and her husband's separation, my mother has seemed sad. She told me that she had been to my father's grave. I wonder if she thinks it's strange that I have never visited my father's grave. I want to do something much more enormous than paying a visit to his grave. When I was talking to my mother, I was wracking my brains trying to think of something new to tell her. I felt devoid of anything at all. I felt like saying, "I can't think of anything to tell you." All I could do was semiautomatically respond to what she was saying. She told me a lot of news. Everything seemed to be fine, but she still sounded sad. It points out that what joy I get out of life is up to me. I can make my life hell or heaven. I felt devoid of any news when talking to my mother, and it was sad talking to her. She's so prompt and punctual about everything, but I would wish her a deeper experience of life somehow. Everything has been a surface or external experience for her, and it almost made motherhood a foreign experience, something hard to understand. The two halves of her life were never unified.

Last night, I was talking to Frank about whether or not to have another baby. What really surprised me is that Frank seems fantastically happy about the pregnancy. Much to my surprise, considering that he'd worked in the basement all day and was tired, he was very understanding. He listened. This morning, at the first sound of the children, he hopped right out of bed, got the children up, fed them, and took them out. At 11:00 a.m. or so, he brought Katherine in and gave her a bottle and put her into bed. So I spent the whole morning in bed. I got myself some toast and coffee, and I was still reading Cooper's *The Death of the Family*. I had the window open in the bedroom and could look over at the green trees and the sunshine and could hear the birds singing. I felt like a completely different person, just being able to stay in bed, and I thought I would very much like to have this baby if I possibly could manage it, and Frank had told me last night that I could get somebody to help me do the housework and that when I came home from the hospital with the baby, I could have a nurse if I wanted one. When I think of that, I think I couldn't ask for anything more than that. That means to me that if I want to have the baby, I can.

I sat in bed this morning, and I thought Katherine did so well with Frank. I wouldn't be afraid to leave her with him for a couple of days. Maybe, I'll take a trip to Boston in September; I could go there for a couple of days. I was thinking of various things and thinking that this time, it would be like having a baby the way I would like to have had Katherine and Thomas, with enough help so that the experience could mean something to me. There would be no point in having the children at all if you don't have time to enjoy them. It was so agonizing, and I was so ill that I couldn't enjoy them. I mean, isn't the whole point of having children, to enjoy them? This time, the third time around, it's going to be perfect; that's something that surprises me. I guess people who get married a lot feel this way—that by the third or fourth marriage, they've perfected it. Or maybe, it's like sex, each time you have a better idea of what to expect: you can then determine things so that you can get what you expect.

The first time you have a baby, it just happens to you. You can decide to have the baby, but the experiences are not quite felt because of the surprise and because you can't anticipate them. Then your second baby helps you recover from the trauma of the first. Then the third one is exactly the way you want it. You're not fooled by what's unimportant. This is what I would have wanted the first time. I wanted to be so happy; I remember, about two months after Katherine was born, I felt either that marrying Frank and having these two children were the dumbest things I ever did or else they were the greatest things I ever did. Of course, now, I'm convinced that it was the greatest. I feel that it was a self-liberating experience. At times though, I can feel so hard-pressed, subhuman, yet at the same time, I think I feel happier than ever before, and I think I am having my own revolution.

Then Frank put leftovers in the oven to heat up for lunch, and while we were having lunch, Frank said, "Why don't you get some new clothes? I mean, how much would it cost to spruce up your wardrobe—$150?" And I said, "Oh yes, that would be fine." What really struck me was that he told me that last night, he dreamed that I left him, that I said, "You know, Frank, this is just too hard," and I left him and the children, and I went and lived with the man next door, and I got a terrific wardrobe—as Frank put it, "a really chic wardrobe"—and I looked great, and this guy had no children. So I said, "How did you feel?" and Frank said, "Well, at first, really bad, and then I got used to the idea." But I kept thinking maybe if Frank dreamed that, he would think, "Free at last, free at last, good God Almighty, free at last." But I didn't tell him that. Instead, I said, "Oh, Frank, thank you so much for letting me stay in bed this morning. I feel like a different person," and Frank said, "You can do the same thing tomorrow."

I feel completely staggered by Frank's being so good to me and then telling me about the dream that he had. I guess that I really do want to have the baby. I think that if it came right to it, you know, killing the baby, I don't think I could do it. I do want to have the baby. It's been this cold and the fact that in the initial part of the pregnancy, I always feel so tired and don't have the right working hormones; things like that get me down, and I feel extremely tired. But now, I feel super motivated in spite of my feelings of tiredness. Partly, I resent the fact that so much of my time is taken up with dumb chores and not spent with the children. I want to spend a lot of time with the children. I want to learn about my children.

This morning, when I was looking out the window, I saw Frank out at the swings with Katherine and Thomas. They're just adorable children, unbelievably adorable, and seeing their hair blowing in the wind, covered with sunshine, was so beautiful. Frank is the most marvelous father.

Last night, Katherine was going through all her tricks for Granddaddy. Where is your hair, your nose, your mouth, your teeth, your fingers, your toes. She knows all of them, and she even distinguishes between her mouth and her teeth, and she can answer these: What does the kitty say? *Meow.* What does the doggie say? *Woof-woof.* What does a duck say? *Quack, quack.* And how big are you? And she lifts up her two hands. Thomas was talking to Granddaddy, and he told him that he didn't like peanut butter very much. Thomas told me, "Granddaddy is awfully ticklish."

Thursday, June 10, 1971

Yesterday, I had an appointment to see Dr. Kuhn. I thought that by June 9, the date of the appointment, I would have made up my mind about whether or not I wanted to have the baby. And so I have. I have made up my mind to have the baby. My reasons for not having it were slight, but I had to consider them and work my way through them: overpopulation, pollution, the fact that it would be such a lot of work for me, and I can hardly do any more than I'm doing now. And I thought about our having so little money. I look at somebody like Rina and Frank Plow. They have three children, and they always seem so absolutely worn-down and so hard-pressed and exhausted that they can hardly manage. I don't want our life to be like that. I don't want Frank to feel that he's just got to grind away and grind away and grind away and that his only purpose in life is to earn money to support this bunch of people. Yet I see that Frank is extremely happy about the baby. He has been so nice to me about it, and he has said, "Do whatever you want, but I think we should have the baby." He said, "What if we aborted this child and then something happened to Katherine or Thomas? We'd probably never have any more, and we'd be left with one child. That would be really sad." Two of my brothers have no children of their own. Frank has a brother who has one child. You might say that just within our family, there are slots. He said we could get somebody to help me and that probably, I should have a nurse when I come home from the hospital. He could hardly do any more than that, and he's assured me that the money situation will get better. Actually, I think he's much happier. Anyway, my reasons for wanting the child are overwhelming, and I wanted it to be a chosen child so that when I'm up all night with the baby, I won't think, "Well, if only this hadn't happened." I asked myself, "Why do I want to have the child?" And it's obvious that I want the child for my own sake—less for the child's sake, mostly for my very own sake. And I think that probably, on a very instinctive level, once a woman has a baby, she always wants a baby. I mean, she yearns for a feeling of completeness; after she has a baby, it seems there is a void there that the birth has created. She wants to fill this void. Naturally, this can be extreme if you have sixteen children, like the woman in the Anne Bancroft movie *Pumpkin Eater*. It can be ridiculous, but on a very basic level, I think there is a strong desire, and it seems even stronger to me now because I'll be thirty-nine years old this July, and this is really my last chance.

There are a couple of other reasons for having another baby. One of them is that I feel I can make something nice of the experience; given another chance, I can do it better, with more grace, than I did with Thomas or with Katherine. Katherine will be two in September, and I feel that I have not gotten as much out of the experience of motherhood as I wanted to. For a year after Thomas was born, I was really in shock, and it was impossible to even talk about the experience. By the time Thomas was a year old, I was already a couple of months pregnant with Katherine, and we bought the house and moved. In both cases, it seemed as though I was gypped out of the experience, but I don't see how the aftermath of Thomas's birth could have been any different. And Katherine was truly a beautiful experience. It was exquisite. How is it that from the time Thomas was born until he was a year old, I was so unhappy, and then from the time that Katherine was born until the time that he was two, I was so happy? Although I was very happy with Katherine, I didn't take any notes on the pregnancy, and I was just barely conscious of the nature of the experience. Now, I want an experience that will be all mine, where I can have it the way I want to, and where I can keep notes on it. Because of the past two experiences, I'm more aware of the nature of the experience, and because of that, I'll be able to say more. If I had written about Katherine and Thomas, maybe that would have made the experiences different. I don't know.

I feel as though I had just ordered a meal, finished the meal, came out the door, hesitated a bit, and turned around and ordered another meal. And I say to myself, "Why did I do that?" Now, I'm going to record what it's like. I won't be so scared that the child is going to die or somehow be abnormal. Maybe, this time, I will be able to create images that will give a picture of the experience. But I don't want the experience of motherhood to be quite over. And the question has always been between two children and three children. So I guess it's better to have three in my case, and I don't think I'll regret it, rather than to have two and perhaps regret it, especially, as Frank said, if anything should happen to Katherine or Thomas.

But I have felt so exhausted. In the early spring, Dr. Rosenberg thought I had mononucleosis, and Katherine is difficult to watch right now. She's climbing, and sometimes, she falls or trips and falls when she goes from the grass to the concrete. She just can't be left alone outside for a minute.

We've had almost no spring, and suddenly, it got very, very hot, and the summer around here, especially here in Kettering, is dull because it's too hot to go out during most of the day. For a couple of days, not even the leaves on the trees moved. Everything seemed desertlike, and I felt a kind of boredom. Katherine's been waking up from her nap, and I think there's almost nothing I can do when she is awake. I do things in the morning, but in the later afternoon, all I can do is watch her, and for long hours. Then I think of going all through this again, and I wonder if I really like being a mother. There are certain stages that I just endure—for instance, there's not a meal that goes by that Katherine doesn't either throw food or dump out her milk. It seems as though some days, I do nothing but clean up endless slop and glop. But I just bear it, and the rewards are great; those things are minor frustrations, nothing more than that. I ask, "What if the child were retarded and would never be any better than that?"

I felt so happy when I was pregnant with Katherine, euphoric. I want to feel that way again. I want to be happy more than anything else. I want to be happy, and I want to be joyful. I want to live this particular period to the fullest. I want to unite the instinctual side of life with the ego side of life, and I think that this is something that women that I have known have failed to do. The only women I know of that are not like this are very creative women, somebody like Käthe Kollwitz or Mary Cassatt. It is because they are creative, because they are giving shape to something. They let out something that's inside them, and I think that the task for women is to unite these two so that ego serves instinct. And if we do, the whole world will be so different. We'll have forms for things that we've never dreamed.

I do feel bad that I never did write much about either of the previous pregnancies, and so that's why I've decided to have the baby, and yesterday, I went to Dr. Kuhn, and I told him that I felt very pregnant, and he said, "You seem to be really quite big, considering the early stage." Maybe, I'll have twins.

We had Thomas with us. Frank, Thomas, and I went to Martin's for lunch, and then we went to the Store and bought some Arabia dishes and some flowers. Then we went and bought a Sony tape recorder and went home. It was a fabulous day, a really fabulous day, just to see the things in the store! Frank saw a shiny black Parsons table, and he said, "Wouldn't that be great for the kitchen?" And it really would be. It's a brilliant idea to have that table for the kitchen.

Now, I'm in such a different frame of mind than in that interim period before one's body gets into the swing of being pregnant. I'm in a wasteland. Everything is dull and empty. I feel as though some hormone is not being produced. I feel slightly bored, and that's the most unusual feeling for me. I almost never feel bored. I do feel anxious to record. For three years, I didn't do anything like that, and I wanted to. In some strange way, it's just as well that I didn't because then I would wonder if I had the experiences I had just to write about them or if I had used these recordings as my escape—what I mean to say is not really responding or not doing housework when the children are asleep, rather doing some recording. But I cannot feel that way because for three years, I didn't do any recording.

I'm beginning to feel happier than I did. For a while, it seemed as though things around me were disintegrating; everywhere I looked at the wall or anywhere, there were marks and marks and marks. Then trying to get the dryer installed, getting draperies, buying more china and endless numbers of things. Things deteriorate faster than I can keep up with them. I look at my closet, and I think the house needs cleaning and a going-over, and to have another baby means that these things are not going to get done soon. I'll have the rest of my life to clean the house, and that's the only way to look at it. I want to do something much more important with this experience. I see now that I'm in a position to do it, one I've never been in before. We're not in the midst of moving, and we're not hammering out what our lifestyle is going to be. I absolutely know now what I want to do, and there are just a few things that bother me. One of them is that Thomas goes out to play now by himself to Freddy and Gregory's home, and several times, their mother, Rina, has fed him. He goes in the house, and they feed him, and Frank said to me, "They'll probably get to know Thomas better than we will." Another irritant is that there's nothing in our backyard to hold the kids' attention, like a pool or sandbox. There's no shade, and to give the kids lunch out there means going out into the heat again and down over a steep hill from our kitchen. There's no exit. I could go down the stairs through the basement, but the basement is unfinished. There's nothing out there like a jungle gym or a swing set. When Thomas goes out, he immediately gravitates down to the Plows. I don't really want him to bother Rina, and I don't really want him to eat down there, but I'm not doing anything to entice the kids up here or to have little sessions up here that they really like. The problems: Thomas goes out, and he takes his bike; then he comes back, no bike, and I have to go out and look for it. Or he goes out to play, and I can't find him, and I look out the window, and I'm carrying Katherine, and she's heavy and she's crying. I look at the neighbors, and they look so much like they're struggling. I think this whole picture of little children in the suburbs and these people that are bringing up their kids in this complete world that doesn't really connect with anything else makes me feel awful. It makes me feel like throwing up as though I have ashes in my mouth and I want to spit them out.

I don't feel threatened by that anymore, but I look at them, and I think, "How do I look in comparison to them?" I probably look worse. Jeannette, my next-door neighbor, works all day long on her house. I get depressed when I look at our neighbors, when I look out and down toward Joyceton Street to the row of little houses during the long hours from about four in the afternoon until nine in the evening. I'm just watching Katherine. I feel that maybe, I'm not a good-enough mother and that I'm not providing enough stimulation for Thomas and his friends. I don't know.

The past couple of weeks, the late afternoons have been difficult. I feel very tired. On top of that, I feel very tired from the pregnancy. I think, maybe, it's too much for me. It's going to be harder to travel and do everything with three. Nevertheless, I still want to have the baby. I was happy yesterday when we got this Sony cassette tape recorder because now, I'll be able to have somebody type the notes that I made previously. That is a big step forward for me.

Frank and I were talking about his father and about his brother Alfred, and I said that I really admired Frank's parents more than Hettie and Alfred. Frank said, "Yeah, but Hettie and Alfred are takers, and my parents are givers." I thought to myself later, "I want to be a giver and not a taker." In spite of whatever Frank does professionally or what we have, I don't want to be mindful only of the things I don't have. I really want to give, and I want to create a beautiful atmosphere.

Anna called this morning. I had a great talk with her about motherhood. It's easier to talk to her than to anybody else, which is really strange. I asked her if she knew of any Jungian things on motherhood, and she said that the best thing that she knew was a talk given by Anne Belford Ulanov, and she suggested that I write to her. She's the woman that Anna told me about previously who said that the birth of the baby is like the birth of spiritual and religious consciousness and that you wouldn't pull on a plant to make it grow. Anna said that her talk was really the best thing she ever heard on motherhood and that Mrs. Ulanov said that the process of individuation is like motherhood. The birth of the self is like the birth of a child. It is a very inward experience although it's also very difficult to get women to talk about it. Anna said that Jung said (about motherhood) women have a task for civilization and that their task is to emphasize the feminine side of life. I am convinced that's true because there would have to be outward forms; first, there are images, and then there are ideas. Women have to create the images, but I don't think they can do it until their ego side and their instinctual side are united. Anyway, it was wonderful to talk to Anna.

With our trip out yesterday and the fact that we are going to have a new baby, getting the tape machine, taping Anna's call, and Frank being so great, I felt so happy. The only other thing that could have happened was the library telling me they had the book I requested. I thought to myself, "These nice experiences should carry me through. I've got to keep sight of the peaks and not get stuck in the valleys."

Tuesday, June 15, 1971

Getting the tape recorder was a major stride. I'll be able to get things typed more easily. After I stop and think about it, I realize that it would be extremely difficult to have anyone here typing in the living room. With two little children and somebody here either at night or during the day when Frank is here, it would be very difficult. Once I get the patch cord and the extra cassettes, I should be ready to go. I appreciate the fact that Frank let me get it, and I also appreciate the fact that Frank told me I could hire somebody to come and help me in the house. I've called some agencies, and I think that I probably will be able to find somebody. That's really going to make a very big difference, an enormous difference. I want to get a couple of babysitters that I can call on quite easily just to come over for a couple of hours in the afternoon. I'd like to have somebody take Katherine Louise out in the late afternoon, but maybe, she's still too young. Last night, I had Katherine out, and she fell on the sidewalk and gave her knee such a scrape. She's still capable of falling so easily going from the grass to the concrete. But I appreciate the fact that Frank's letting me get someone to help with the housework every other week and also the recorder and the fact that he will pay to have some of these recordings typed.

I still, from time to time, ask myself if I really want to have a baby, and I guess that I do want to have the baby.

My day at the present time is more or less in two shifts, like working from 7:00 a.m. to 3:00 p.m. and then from 3:00 p.m. to 11:00 p.m., two eight-hour shifts with usually, but not always, a little break in between. To live without satisfying any of the demands of your individual self is impossible. From about 4:00 p.m., when Katherine wakes up from her nap, I wait a few minutes and give her a chance to wake up, and I usually wash my face as though I'm getting myself ready for the next stint. I've asked myself, "Do I really love her, and do I really want to have another baby?" and then I go in to get her in the crib, and I say, "Hello, Katherine, did you wake up from your nap?" I pick her up and hold her, and I just love her so much that the previous reluctance goes away, and I realize that without little Katherine to pick up when she wakes up from her nap, that time to myself would be meaningless. On the other hand, without any time to myself at all, my life would be maybe not totally meaningless, but almost meaningless. One really enhances the other although there's a slight lump in my throat as I transfer from one to the other.

Lately, on that second shift, I have felt exhausted. I've felt too tired to take Katherine out. I get the children up from their naps, and I know there's going to be hours of watching them. I try to play with them and do a certain amount of things with them. But oh, Thomas hits Katherine sometimes, or she wants to go out, or else she's up at the sink or climbing on something she isn't supposed to be on, and I have to watch her every single minute. In the house, she's almost at the end of that phase, and I can leave her in the room with Thomas for a minute and not feel that he might hit her. I used to feel that he just might hit her or poke out her eye. I don't feel that way now. He might give her a shove, but not the kind of thing where he'd push her over and she'd hit her head and be unconscious. That afternoon stretch though is something to endure. I usually don't know what time Frank will be home for dinner. I used to wonder whether to wait for him or not. Now, the thing is to eat at six and then take the children out afterward. By then, it will be a little bit cooler.

For the past weeks, around 5:00 p.m., I feel exhausted; I can hardly get anything to eat, or I can hardly change the children's pants or take them out. It is standing, standing, watching Katherine, and standing every minute. She likes to go up to the swings, but I have to stand in such an awkward position to swing her because I have to hold on to her at the same time because I can't quite trust that she, by herself, will hold on, and I've got to keep her away from a swing that's in motion. She likes to go up on the slide, but she has to be held as she climbs up to the top of the slide. All this has made me wonder if I really want another baby, yet I know I do. I don't know how I'll get through the work involved in it. If only I can find someone to help. Katherine was born just a couple of weeks after we moved here, and I didn't know anyone that would babysit then. This time, it will be different. I feel so much that I have come into my own. It's like knowing how to work the system, like knowing how to use whatever advantages and resources a place has to offer.

I was looking through some notebooks in the drawer. I was tying to find if I had written anything before or after Thomas was born besides

35

the notes that I kept, if I had written anything in the diary from the time he was born until the time that we moved here. I saw that I finished my motherhood piece, and I remembered that the first year was so unhappy, the second year so happy. I was thinking that either I'll add a chapter to the motherhood piece, or I'll do another piece, which is in addition to this diary that I'm keeping now on the pregnancy.

As I was looking through my notebooks, I came upon notes I made about a conversation that my friend Emily and I had a few months before Thomas was born. Emily said to me, "Gee, Katherine, why don't you quit your job?" And I said, "Why do you say that, Emily? Do you think it's too much for me? Why do you say that?" It was very strange reading this. Emily said, "Because I think you could make such a nice experience of it. You cook now, but you could sew, and you could probably make something more of your experience in Hyattsville." I didn't think of it consciously in these terms, but when I look back, I felt very threatened when Emily said that because I felt that she thought physically, I was barely able to work during my pregnancy. Maybe, she thought my heart really wasn't in my job or that I wasn't doing a good job. It's similar to when I got married. It seemed to me that my friends were so happy when I got married that it made me suspicious. Did they think that I wasn't professionally that good? Didn't they think that I was going to be a loss to the profession if I didn't continue to work? When Emily said that, it was the same thing again. She said, "I think you can make something so nice of the experience." It was similar to the time before Thomas was born. I worked like absolutely mad on that bibliography. I had finished the body of it, and the indexes were still hanging fire, but after he was born, there were innumerable phone calls back and forth about one thing or another about the bibliography and the indexes and what should be done with the indexes and what could be done with them and what would be the fate of the bibliography. Before Thomas was born, I never gave what was happening any thought so that it was like—*crash*—all of a sudden, there was a baby. In the apartment, before he was born, I worked sixteen hours a day on that bibliography. I wanted so much to finish it because I felt guilty about not fulfilling my obligation. Also, I had the drive to complete something, and I didn't want to lose what had been done so far. It seemed that I would be able to finish it before the baby was born, and that's what I wanted to do because if I didn't, I felt that all of it might just go down the drain.

When I think about having this baby though, I think I can make such a nice experience of it. That's why I want to have it. And it can be all the things that my pregnancy with Thomas was not. And it can be the things that my pregnancy with Katherine was, which I never did get the time to make notes about. It can be a repetition of ecstasy, and now that I know the nature of that experience, I want to record it. I can appreciate this in a way that I just could not appreciate Thomas's birth and that I almost appreciated during Katherine's birth, but not 100 percent. I want to drink the experience of motherhood right to the very bottom of the cup. I want to see everything that's in it. We are here in this house. We have the setting. This should really be my baby, not the doctor's or anybody else's.

I was reading something in that *Child Equals One* book, which said that by the time a child is three, which is how old Thomas is, his whole personality is formed. I think that's amazing. I just wonder, if I could do it all over again with Thomas, what I would have done differently. I don't know what else I could have done, but looking at that *Equals One* magazine that Anna sent me, with the issue on the child, that's the kind of thing I never looked at before Thomas was born. I did get a couple of books out of the library about what happens during the development of the child at ten weeks, at twenty weeks, and so forth. But I really didn't have anything else.

Everything just changed so fast on that November day when I started bleeding; from then on, I was confined to bed rest in the apartment. I did have on order at the Trover Shop on Capitol Hill several books by Harding, one by Wickes, and one by Bertine. It was the last gesture I made before I was completely confined. It was all so abrupt. This time, it's different.

I was reading an article in *Mademoiselle* by Hortense Calisher called "The House." She says there's "in" and there's "out," and there are "foreground" women and "background" women, although the "background" women are pretty much extinct. But you know, this "in" and "out" thing, the symbol for this is the house. The women are pointed, like beagles, to "out" and live their lives that way, or else, they are pointed to "in," and even though the choice is really unconscious on the women's part, it's the defining thing in her life, and sooner or later, she does get a house, no matter what she calls it.

When I see something like that, I think of cleaning my room when I was ten years old and the way that I felt about my childhood home and the way that I have always felt about every place that I have lived in and how my life has been a search for the perfect home.

There were places that I used to see when I walked from MIT to the subway at Kendall Square; there were offices that I used to walk by, and I used to look into the offices and think, "How can they find anybody to work in there?" They are so unbelievably awful. I didn't even like to walk past them. It was the same with places I used to see where people lived. Probably, the most awful thing, it seemed to me, was what if I had to live in a place like that, some place I hated. I used to always think of finding the perfect home. Eventually, I thought when we moved here that you don't find it, you create it. You make it yourself. And then you never have to be afraid. No one can ever take it from you because you can start building it all over again. In fact, to have it really be yours, to feel that you can really relate to it as an environment, as a kind of outer shell to yourself, you really have to create it yourself.

Our family home could have been completely different, even though that wasn't the most fascinating neighborhood that you could imagine. I think that is probably true of this house. Connie said to me when I told her I was marrying Frank and I said I didn't think I could stand to live where he wanted to live, "Well, that's crazy. You should be able to make a home anywhere." But when I finally came around to that point of view, it was Connie who came here and said, "These kind of houses just don't do anything for my imagination. They really don't turn me on at all." I had asked her what she could suggest we could do to this house, and she said she couldn't think of anything and that she wouldn't spend any money on this house at all. She would move out as soon as possible. It reminds me of when I read Lillian Hellman's book. She mentioned that when she was married and living in Hollywood, she didn't realize how much she hated the place where she lived. I think that when you hate the place where you live, you cannot relate to your deepest self. What makes the difference here is that I can look across the street at trees. Sometimes, it all looks so ethereal, like a Chinese landscape, especially when it's very cloudy. In the morning, when the sunlight hits the trees, it looks one way, and in the evening, another. In the autumn, it looks so different from winter. There is life and drama and constant change. I might have felt the same way about this house as Lillian Hellman did about hers if it didn't have those trees across the street. I don't know what's going to happen if they cut them down. I am told that is what is planned. I guess, maybe, I'll be braver by then. I don't know. What sustains me now are the trees across the street.

I can remember a couple of times writing something about the trees, the house, myself, and then showing it to Connie, and Connie saying, "You should try to recreate reality and have a plot and characters." I just noticed that now and realize that the whole thing isn't for me. Even reading the Hortense Calisher article, I don't even know if it's fiction or nonfiction or if it's excerpted from a couple of things, but it's written in the style I like to write in. My style is probably plainer, but it is like a personal essay. There's conversation if you want to have conversation and references to things that may not be true.

I feel that the Women's Liberation Movement is behind me, and so many things have happened that are fascinating and make the world more interesting and exciting. I guess this baby means that I'm going to be all that much deeper into life and into its problems, and so much has happened in the world that hadn't happened when I was expecting Thomas. And that's part of why I want to have another baby. I find in the Women's Liberation Movement so much more support for the things I feel and I would like to say. This thing about the house, for instance; it isn't even so much what Hortense Calisher said, but it's important to me that something on this subject could get printed because before, when I talked to anybody about such things, it was like telling someone you wet the bed at night, as if you were confiding some shameful or pitiful secret. I have much more of a vision now of what I want, and it's partly because we are in this house, I see a little better what our lifestyle is, and I feel that I have a place here. And I have the support to do what I think I want to do and a vision of what I want to do. Maybe, the thing about the Women's Movement is what Hortense says: women should have a choice between "in" or "out." But the Women's Movement doesn't offer any choice: it's got to be "out." That's because revolutions don't offer choices.

I consider myself an "out" who has just transferred "in," and "in" is really only meaningful if you've first been "out"; otherwise, you're too close to it, too much a part of the process yourself. It has to do with consciousness. If you've been "out" and you've transferred "in," then you're more conscious and more aware. You've got the awareness, the language, the voice to express something where you would probably otherwise be inarticulate, silent even to yourself. After women go through "out," because they are forced to, then "in" will take on a whole different meaning. But I do think that the problem at hand for women is to unite ego and instinct. If that's not done, I guess this civilization will die. There has to be more cultural forms for healing, helping, and supporting people.

We told Frank's parents about the baby Sunday night after we came back from Arena Theatre, where we saw the *Sign in Sidney Brustein's Window*. They acted very strange about it, maybe a little as though it was something to be ashamed of. They said something like "Try to be happy about it because it might not work out very well," as if Frank and I are somehow wrong or inept. It was so interesting to hear this from Anna: when I said, "Well, when I've talked to some women who have had babies, asked them questions, it seems that they don't have the thoughts or feelings or experiences that I have," Anna said, "A lot of people have lived their whole lives and haven't experienced their lives the way you experience yours." I'd like to ask her how she thinks I've experienced my life. That raises such an interesting question. I was thinking about that man on TV who teaches at George Washington University and had that one-to-one program where he was a literary critic. I used to wonder if he experienced his life differently from the way other people experienced theirs.

One of the things in Cooper's the *Death of the Family* that intrigued me was that he said some people go through their whole lives feeling that their lives are directed from outside. I guess that's one of the things that I really appreciate about my life: I feel that my life is directed from the inside. I feel that almost everything that happens to me happens because I want it to happen. Sometimes, I bite off a little more than I can chew, but I think my life is what I want it to be. Maybe, that's my biggest illusion. I can't blame anybody for my life. I can see that my life is the way I want it to be, to some extent, because of my mother, but I had to have had some mother. I suppose that when women can unite their instinctual sides and their ego sides, the whole human race will realize that life should be directed more from the inside. That is when the person matures and has been born a self.

Frank told me that one Saturday, Lesley Branck came into his office. Her two-year-old child died not long ago. He got into a fish pond somewhere in the backyard and drowned. Frank said Lesley was extremely gracious and that she looked very nice. She said that if she didn't have their little nine-month-old, she doesn't know how they'd go on. She told Frank that the grief is a feeling you cannot express to anybody. Frank said that he thought that she would probably get pregnant right away again. I thought, "Would I have been better off if I worked in the library?" because I think that you have to think of yourself as a person as well all the time.

Friday, June 18, 1971

Within a small range, it's so hard to predict and plan things with the children. Yesterday morning, we went to the Y to register the two children for swimming classes. When we came back, I put the children in for their naps, and Katherine never took a nap. I'd get her up and put her back and get her up and put her back. It seemed stupid, all the effort for nothing. Today, on the other hand, I put her in for a nap, and she's still sleeping. I tried to wake Thomas up so that he could watch *Sesame Street*; I roused him a little bit, but he just went back to sleep, and he's still asleep now. There were about twenty-five people standing in line at the Y yesterday. Frank and I took turns standing in line although Frank stood in line most of the time and I sat down. And some of the time, I held Katherine, and some of the time, he held Katherine. It's awfully hard for me to stand, and when I was at the Y, I kept thinking, "It's almost frightening when I try to do anything like this: getting up, getting breakfast, getting the two kids and myself dressed, and all of us into the car. Just being on my feet for any length of time is exhausting. That, plus the fact that I feel such bladder pressure and such an urge to urinate that unless the ladies room is handy, I begin to feel worried. On a day like yesterday, when Katherine just never slept, by the end of the afternoon, I feel worn down, and that's when I begin to ask myself, "Can I handle another baby?" With Katherine's fussing at this difficult age, taking her out and standing and standing and following her all around, it makes me wonder.

This morning, I got breakfast, and Frank left for work. Katherine coughed a tremendous lot last night. She has a bad cold. We all have colds although I'm better today, but Katherine just coughed and coughed. I took her temperature this morning, and she didn't have a fever, but I was going to call Dr. Molning anyway. I got the children dressed, cleared away the breakfast things, and put away some of the clean dishes. I wanted to vacuum before calling Dr. Molning and then taking the children out. It must have been quarter to eleven or so before I got them out, and no sooner had I gotten them out than Katherine fell down on the concrete and scraped her knee, not very badly, but she cried, and I brought her in, and I put mercurochrome on her knee, and she cried and cried. And while she was crying, Frank's mother called; then we went out again, and Thomas kept pulling the wire that comes out of the inside of the house and connects with the water meter, and I said, "No, no, Thomas. No, no." Then he went over, and he was going to turn on the faucet, and I said, "No, no, Thomas. No, no." Then he had this trowel, which was by a flower pot, that Frank had used to plant the azaleas. It's probably not too dangerous for Thomas, but it is dangerous for Katherine, so I said, "Thomas, give me that." Of course, he ignored me. It's hard to imagine that he could get into that many things so fast. I didn't mean to seem annoyed with him, but it seems that it's such a job not just to watch him, but to do something that's fun and constructive with him. Not too long afterward, Thomas said that he wanted something to drink, and he wanted to come in; it was getting close to noon, so I gave them their lunch, and Katherine just dumped her whole lunch on the floor, and then she started to cry and kept crying, and I assumed that she must have been tired. So I made up her bottle and put her into bed, and Thomas watched *Sesame Street*, and I sat out in a chair for a short time. Then Frank's office called and asked if he should pick up a prescription. I figured he would be home, and I thought, "Well, we've had our lunch. I'll just sit out here and relax a little bit, and if he comes, okay, and if he doesn't come, okay, but it does bother me to wait for him to come home for a meal, or if I go ahead and eat and then he turns up afterward, I'm put off." Anyway, I thought I wouldn't let it bother me. When he came along, he got out of the car and started raking up the lawn. After about half an hour, he said, "What's for lunch?" I said that there were a lot of things, like liverwurst, ham, or salad. Then he said, "Here I am waiting all this time for lunch and you've already eaten!" He was so hurt, and Katherine was crying in her crib, and *Sesame Street* was almost finished, so I got her up, and it was just as well so that I could give her some more medicine. I brought her out in the kitchen. Thomas wanted milk. He had his milk, and he spilled his milk. Then he wanted a sandwich, so I gave him the makings of a sandwich, and he said, "Not this, not this, not that, no, I want to do it." Katherine dumped out her milk, and then Frank said, "Do you think that I can have cake without them wanting it?" So I said, "Why don't you give them a little cake?" So there were crumbs everywhere. I mopped up the floor and mopped up the floor and mopped up the floor. The children are one thing, but when Frank also turns up and he is really hurt that we had our lunch already, that's another. Finally, I put the two children in for naps, and they both went right to sleep, and they are still asleep. So it turned into a lovely afternoon.

I went outside and sat in the sun. I had been feeling so exhausted that I felt I was on the verge of an exhaustive collapse. I think it's mainly the pregnancy, but there is the fact that Dr. Rosenberg thought I had mono at the beginning of the year. I decided then that I was going to try to take it as easy as I possibly could. Frank says I shouldn't think of things I do as work, but I go about from 7:00 a.m. to 3:00 p.m. and then from 3:00 p.m. to 11:00 p.m. By the time I get Thomas into bed, make some coffee, pick up some of the toys or the clothes that are scattered all around, run downstairs to hang up that wash that I didn't get a chance to do all day, or sweep the kitchen floor so there won't be any ants there, it is always about eleven. Sometimes, Thomas gets into bed at ten, but it seems too hard to get him into bed by the time he gets into his pajamas and after he's been read to, does a drawing, and has a drink. It may be eight in the morning before the children wake up, but it's really like working two shifts in one day, and it's hard to feel refreshed and restored in the morning because I'm so tired and my energy is so low. It's so easy to lose patience with the children. I have this vision of how I want to be so loving toward them and, above all, be stimulating to them, to do things with them that are fun, to play games with them all the time. But just to get them up in the morning, feed them, dress them, then clean up after them is no small task when you're pregnant and tired from the day before.

Today, when Frank left, he said, "I hope you make it through the afternoon." I was angry because it was as though he wanted to annoy me. He can say, "Chin up," or "Think happy," or something like that and I feel my gorge rising in a way that used to happen only with my old boss, Mr. Wenstrum. I was trying to put my finger on what it was, the way that mechanism works. It was the same process with Mr. Wenstrum. If there was an emergency and you said to him, "Mr. Wenstrum, I'll stay late tonight after hours and work on this and catch up," he would say, "Sometimes, you are going to have to stay late, and you're going to have to work on this." He would say it as if I hadn't first said it myself. "The chief would agree with me on this, and I'm not sure he will be too pleased." He would accuse you of what you had already admitted and were trying to remedy. If it was a typing correction, he'd say, "This isn't too good. This isn't too good. I don't think that this is going to pass." When you'd say, "I'll correct it," he'd go on and on and on until finally, you felt like saying, "I'm not going to do anything. That's just tough." I would feel like hitting him over the head.

I had decided beforehand that I have two schedules. I ate, and the kids ate, and then Frank came home. When Frank was leaving, Katherine had gotten out of her high chair. She had reached up to the table and got the liverwurst, which had mayonnaise smeared on both sides, out of Thomas's sandwich, and she came into the living room with it to wave goodbye to Frank. Of course, she dropped a piece of it on the floor, so there's mayonnaise and liverwurst from the window to the kitchen table and on to the living room window. Then there's a double set of meals. I guess I should figure it's nice that the children see Frank because the children's day has so little stimulation that it is nice for them to see him. And as it worked out, it was just as well that she didn't go to sleep when I first put her into her crib because then she got some of her medicine and she had a better sleep. She coughed very, very little, and she'll probably feel a lot better when she wakes up. In the end, it all worked out all right, but it's during times like this that I think, "Am I totally mad to have another baby?"

Frank was telling me about the chief pathologist at the Prince George's County Hospital. He owns three farms—one in Pennsylvania, one in Virginia, and one in Maryland. For one of the farms, he paid $450,000. That makes me think we're really poor. I never felt poor before I was married, before I lived in this community. I wonder if I would do anything differently if we had more money. I don't think so. I'd get someone to clean the house, and I'd try to be more rested, more fun, and more cheerful all the time with the children. I guess they have to accept the fact that I'm human too and understand that I try to do the best that I can. I might have slightly better clothes. I don't think the children would be any different. I don't think they'd be any better than they are now. I'd want to have the children just as they are. Sometimes, I get so tired that it's just plain scary because I feel weak, and it's frightening to feel weak. But there are moments that are truly sublime, and I blame those other feelings on my being close to exhaustion, and there are always moments that are terribly trying with little children. There are moments that are absolutely sublime, such as when I get up very early in the morning and go out with a cup of coffee on the front step while everybody is still sleeping. I have an overwhelming urge to meditate, to reflect, to daydream.

When I eat with Katherine and she's in her high chair, she's almost impossible. She's hanging out of her chair, she wants to climb on the table, she cries for things that she can't have, and she's only good in her high chair for about a second. It's torture just to sit at the table and eat with her.

This afternoon, I sat outside in the sun. First, I sat in the sun until that began to feel too hot, and then I moved the chair around to the back, and I sat out in the back under the shade for a while, and then I came in the house, and I took a little nap for half an hour. I slept. Then I got up, and I decided I'd have my evening meal now by myself, when it would really be relaxing, and I would be ready for the children when they wake up. So

I made a sandwich and some tea. It's very peculiar, but I find that when I sleep for half an hour or so in the afternoon, I wake up feeling nauseated. I don't know why I don't feel nauseated in the morning. I guess it's probably because my stomach is empty of food, but if it's really close to my lunchtime when I wake up, I feel dizzy and nauseated and also hungry at the same time, and the only thing that I can do is eat.

I'm going to try to lose some weight because I should weigh at delivery time what I weigh now. I should not gain any more weight at all. Anyway, I got up and had a sandwich and some tea and was sitting there, and it was one of those moments that are truly sublime. The moments that are trying are not deeply that trying, they don't trouble me, but after six glasses of spilled milk, I feel like screaming. What happens to me is that I've lost patience, and I'm worn down to a nub. Then I begin to feel like an animal. As more and more glasses of milk get spilled, I feel as though I'll start banging my head on the floor and work myself into a temper tantrum. I feel so frustrated that I feel like acting the way children do. I can see why little children cry a lot—because they are so frustrated—and when you are with them a lot, you feel the same way that they do. I was reading *Equals One*, the magazine dedicated to wholeness, their special issue on children, which Anna sent me. It stated that by the time a child is three, his character is completely formed. It also says that child prodigies are usually just average children whose mother played with them a lot and that up until the child is six years old, he should be constantly stimulated, and that by the time he's seven, he should have learned any languages and all the sports that he's going to learn. The article also said that children are using only a small portion of their brains—99 percent of the brain is not being used—and that we are artificially retarded by our families and our school system. I read that, and I think I should be doing much, much more for Thomas, and for Katherine too. I'm doing so little.

But these houses! This house in particular! There's so much that should be done, and I do so little. These houses are hard to keep clean. They are new houses, but they're incredibly dusty; the heating system throws out dirt. They seem to be designed to keep women working all the time. I cannot do that. The little bit that I do—the dishes, the laundry, the vacuuming—I detest, but I have to continue doing to keep life going. We have to have clean dishes, and we have to have clean clothes. But I even find that this much housework is a strain on me and leaves me with no energy or time to play with the kids. They are not getting enough mothering, not the right sort, and after reading that article, I began to wonder if we should begin to reconsider sending Thomas to the Montessori school. Would the stimulation and environment that they have outweigh the fact that he's got to be pressured into getting ready in the morning? He'd have to be woken up and be told, "Eat, eat, eat," and "Come on now, get dressed." He'd be on a schedule for five days a week. Would it be better if he dallied around at his own pace, went to preschool maybe two days a week, and then watch *Sesame Street* to stay closer to me? I do so little, and these communities offer nothing, absolutely nothing. It's maddening because I can't even get the help I need for myself to give the children something. Sometimes, I feel so used up that there isn't anything else for me to give. I am literally unable to stand up. And that's when I think, "Should I have another baby?" Maybe, I should concentrate on stimulating the two children that I already have.

I am convinced that the educational system that we have now is just something to get us to function in a job. In the Industrial Revolution, as it now stands, whatever the particular state of the Industrial or Scientific Revolution, that particular state demands people of a certain kind of education, and that's all we have, and that's all we are stimulated for. I want so much more for Katherine and Thomas, but I don't know if they would get any more from me if we didn't have another baby.

Frank got me the tape recorder, and he said that I could have a typist and that I could get a cleaning lady and a sitter to take Katherine out in the afternoon for a walk. I can't expect any more from him than that. He really is a much better parent than I am. I do think that. He has a much better relationship with Thomas than I do. He's a tremendous parent.

Last Wednesday, Frank and his father went to Baltimore, where Frank had an appointment to look at some dental equipment. It was funny because Frank was telling me Thursday morning about the trip, and it's just so typical and so funny. There was a detour in the road, so they lost their way. They had to get off the main highway, and then they couldn't find their way back to it. They went through this absolutely beautiful countryside, and Frank just couldn't believe it was Baltimore. There was a beautiful road with trees on the side, neat farmhouses, and rolling hills, and it was absolutely idyllic. Frank said his father was terribly nervous because they were late for the appointment, so Frank said, "Look at the scenery." Frank's father likes to plan and keep his eye on the goal and just go *zoomph* right to the goal. Frank said his father doesn't enjoy the process. So I said, "Well, Frank, it's almost frightening that you enjoy the process so much; you plan, and you enjoy the process, and you have a desire toward its conclusion, but I think your love for the process is so great that you dissolve into the process." Like the time he asked his parents to come over at ten in the morning to watch the children and they came over about ten minutes past ten o'clock—they were so upset because they were late, and Frank wasn't even dressed yet. Eventually, Frank got dressed. I was ready and waiting. Katherine went in for her nap, and Thomas was with his grandparents. Finally, we leave, go out to get into the car, but Frank and his father take a look at the roof, and they start talking about a shingle that's loose. Frank's mother said to Frank's father, "Don't talk to him now. He's got to get going." And his mother said to me, "How can you stand it? How can you stand it?"

I remember the day that Katherine was christened, and I said, "Oh, Frank, please don't be late," and Frank's mother said to me, "Well, don't tell him like that. Just tell him. Lay the law down to him, you know, get going." Then she told me how whenever they went to mass, she would always be ready half an hour before them and then push and push and push. And she said, "You know, Frank and Dad are just the same. Everything left to the last minute." Almost every time they come over, it's like that. And they are always telling Frank, "Hurry up, hurry up, you'll be late, you'll be late." Many times they've been here and Frank's supposed to go to work at one o'clock, they always keep saying, "Hurry up, you'll be late, you'll be late." Frank doesn't care that he's going to be late. He's never concerned that he'll late. There's so much pressure on him all the time it seems his life is a reaction against it. As a result, he's always late for everything.

I've been wondering about the term "birth of the self." I wonder how old a person is when he's finally born into selfhood. It must be somehow similar to the time after adolescent rebellion when you have forgiven your parents and integrated what they represent into yourself. I suppose that it could happen around age twenty-one. I don't think it could happen before that. Nature is designed so that it happens, like parenthood, or it should happen, like parenthood. In reading this issue of *Equals One* on the child, it stresses the tremendous importance of the mother. In a primitive society, it says that it's not superstition that keeps the mother from never leaving her child during the first two or three years of life. I remember Ellen Moloy saying the same thing about that book that I was never able to get hold of, James Maloney's *Fear, Contagion, and Conquest.* In some primitive societies, from the time of birth until the age of two, the child is never physically separated from the mother's body. The mother carries it on her back or in the front all the time and sleeps by it. In primitive societies, until the time that the child is about three, the mother never leaves it so that it never goes through a separation trauma. The separation at birth is overcome by the closeness to the mother. Women in the United States are so directed to "out" and the possibilities of "out." That is why so many suburban housebound mothers are unhappy, and the world desperately needs mothers and healers at home and needs people who appreciate the quality of existence rather than accomplishments. Women here in the United States just want to get out. That was truer in my lifetime, but that's probably not true for the world. I don't know. You can really only appreciate "in" after you've been "out" because you are only conscious of it after you've been "out."

June 24, 1971

I am so filled with fury. I don't know whether it's fury or resentment or hate. I feel like railing against my environment. I keep telling myself that this probably means it's only me that I'm dissatisfied with. But it seems to me that my life at the present time is really intolerable. I think that it is this way because it's so extremely passive. I think that you feel this way when you're taking care of little children.

But this morning, the children were both awake and jumping up and down in their cribs by seven-thirty, and we got up. I find it difficult to try to do anything, except watch them when they are up. We had breakfast, the usual spilled milks and minor disasters like Thomas is telling Katherine to sit down in her high chair and she continues to stand so he goes over as though he's going to make her sit down. So when we finished eating, Katherine climbs up on the table and tries to empty the salt and pepper shaker everywhere. I just rush to get these things out of her hands, and no sooner can you turn around that she's into something else.

Just to get the dirty dishes into the dishwasher and the clean ones out is difficult because Katherine is always attempting to crawl into the dishwasher. She's crying for attention, and I'm trying to finish up so that I can give her some attention, but with getting breakfast, getting the children dressed, doing a load of washing, vacuuming, doing some straightening up, it's just about impossible to do any housekeeping with the children. I know I don't give the children enough. I don't service their needs. Each morning and each afternoon should really be a session, maybe not exactly like kindergarten, but it should be a session of some sort. We should go out and have fun, either play in the pool in the backyard or go for a walk. It seems almost amazing that my two children are up for so many hours—and they are so lively—from about seven-thirty in the morning until about eleven at night. Today, for instance, I put Katherine in for her nap. It must have been one-thirty in the afternoon, or maybe quarter to two. She went right to sleep. Then I put Thomas in for his nap, and he was talking and making a lot of noise, and I think he woke Katherine up. At any rate, she was awake about forty-five minutes after she went in for her nap. She was awake and ready to get up before Thomas had gone to sleep. That means I don't get any time to myself in the afternoon. When she woke up from her nap, I thought, "What am I going to do with her?" She's into everything imaginable. Watching her and making sure she doesn't get hurt takes hours and hours and hours. She's hard to watch outside because she goes up to the sandbox and gets sand in her eyes, she cannot really get on the swings by herself—not to mention that she doesn't know enough to keep away from swings that are in motion—and she doesn't know enough not to go into the street. There's nothing really in the backyard to hold her attention. Now that we have the kiddie pool out there, maybe that will make a difference.

It just seems that with the little bit of housekeeping that I do and the fact that the children need constant watching for such long hours, I feel so drained that I don't have much more to give them. For almost a week, since last Friday or Saturday, I have been sick with the most awful, and I mean really awful, sore throat. It has been absolutely murder. The glands in my neck were all swollen. Monday, I called Dr. Kuhn. I was just lying in bed, and it was such an agony to swallow. My temperature was about 100°F. He prescribed penicillin, and I've been taking that. Meanwhile, trying to get some rest is no small feat. What with being sick, trying to watch the children, and keeping a minimum of order in the house, my patience is worn thin.

For some reason, in the past week or so, I have become fed up with this area. I think it is probably because I'm sick, but when I look out my kitchen window, I want to throw up in the sink. In these little boxes that people live in, the thing that really bothers me most is that it's so hard to watch the children outside. There's nothing outside, and it's so hot here in the summertime. You can just die. You have to take the children out, and you go out, and there's nothing, absolutely nothing around. It is life with little children and then one other adult, your husband. And other than that, it's really isolation. It's like being under house arrest. The thing that has saved my life up to now is the fact that there are trees across the street. Recently, even the trees in this fantastic heat, I guess because there's no movement in them, they seem less interesting. When the children have both fallen asleep in the afternoon and I try to take a nap, my throat is so sore I can't sleep. When I get up, I feel nauseated, and the house is such a mess—everything is grimy and ticky-tacky. The house needs cleaning.

When I look out at Rina Plow's and Jeannette's houses and all their backyards and these people out in their backyards, I feel that the quality of the environment, the quality of life, is so lacking in texture or color or character. The quality of life here is really very poor. It's so poor that if a woman's job is to give a feeling of richness to existence, as compared to success and accomplishment and goals, I don't really know how she can do it in a place like this. Plus, these houses are very hard to take care of. You have all this grass and practically no trees. Even going out in the car, the only place that's worth going to is the library in Upper Marlboro. Other than that, it's just supermarkets. It's a completely impoverished environment.

I used to think that the trouble with having an environment that is exciting and stimulating and beautiful and rich is that you are so agog at the environment that you don't ever go inward to create anything yourself. You stand there and respond to the environment. I used to think that I really could make something beautiful out of this life. There are some people who could be under house arrest and, as Connie would say, make a beautiful poem out of it. Or a novel. I always felt glad that I could be at home with the children. If I worked, in addition to all these things, with my responsibilities in the house and my responsibilities to the children, there would be all these other things—if it were possible to find time to work, then certainly it would be possible to find the time to write. What better time?

For such a long time, I lived with people who had Gyorgy Kepes's paintings on their walls. I have seen the beautiful things that come out of these people's souls. It's time for me to do something now. I have had every advantage. It's finally time for me to create something myself. I should feel that I don't have the distractions that would come with a tremendously interesting environment. I don't have to run down to the gallery or run down to the bookstore. I can use this period of isolation for writing. I'm beginning to notice it now that the children are big enough to go out—to be in some place like Bearskin Neck, to take them for a walk, or take them to the ocean. I have to watch them anyhow, so I might as well take them someplace that is stimulating for them and for myself too. You could go to the supermarket forever here, and you'd never meet anyone else that you knew. In a smaller, scaled-down-to-human-terms setting, you'd probably , have a chance to see people when you are out.

I would expect that my inner life would sustain me during this time; it did here in Kettering. It has up to now, to about a week ago, and I don't know whether it's the drain on me because of the pregnancy or the combination of being pregnant and having this horrible sore throat and the extreme difficulty I have watching the children for the hours and hours and hours that they are up, and there is nothing for them. It's not just me. I could spin something from myself, but I don't know why it should suddenly start bothering me, but it did. I just look out the window and I want to vomit. I have so little time for myself, and now, when I put the children in for a nap and Katherine's awake in her crib, fussing to get up, and it's so fantastically hot to go out for a couple of hours, I just feel sick. The strange thing is that I keep telling myself that I have made what I think of as several strides forward. I do have an agency trying to get me a cleaning woman, I'm also going to try to get a babysitter to take Katherine out in the afternoon, I think I have a typist lined up, and I sent down to Fidelity Sound for a patch cord that would make it possible to duplicate tape from the Tanberg to the Sony cassette recorder. All these things are strides forward.

I was reading a review of a book by Elizabeth Janeway called *Man's World, Woman's Place*. The review was by Margaret Mead in the *New York Times*. She talked about the myth of a woman's place being in the home and how this myth has grown up since suburbia and the rise of the Victorian middle class. Mead mentioned the fact that women are supposed to play three roles simultaneously: mother, housekeeper, and wife. Men, however, are expected to be just one thing at a time; they weren't expected to practice dentistry, for example, and watch the children too. She said it was no wonder a lot of young people are turning to drugs because all they know is the emotions of a modern suburban home, and they have no contact with the real world. The more I think about it, the more I begin to think that maybe, I'm doing the children more harm than good by staying here. It's a strange, completely isolated life. The price you pay for safety is solitary confinement.

We bought some dishes at the Store, and they have discontinued selling the size of the dinner plate that we started getting. I feel so much that what I do depends on Frank, especially the way he's got our finances set up, so that buying these dishes and other things is always done in dribs and drabs, and every time I go back to get more of them, they have discontinued selling them. I feel so fed up with everything—at the rate at which Frank is working on the downstairs, and the downstairs is so filthy, filled with concrete dust. It comes upstairs every time someone comes up, and he doesn't have the dryer hooked up for me yet. Instead of being annoyed with him, I thought I should carve out some little area for myself and, like what the furniture maker George Nakashima said, find some little space somewhere and start creating cells.

To be near the ocean in this weather, to have a walk along the ocean, or to have someplace to walk with the children to would be wonderful. But

I look out and look out back from the kitchen, and I see this little row of boxes. I taste ash on my tongue and feel the dryness in my throat. Maybe, that's what caused my illness, looking out the window. But I don't need a stimulating environment myself, as long as I get a little time to myself. I don't see any other people, and the couple of neighbors that are around here I don't feel any particular desire to talk to. They seem boring to me.

The amount of work that the house requires is fantastic. We are going to have to get a storm window for the living room because when Frank put the humidifier in, the window fogged up so much that the moisture began to destroy the wallboard under the window. And the paint on the shutters outside is flaking off, so we will have to paint them. We have a lawnmower that practically doesn't work; Frank is taking care of the lawnmower that doesn't work, his two automobiles that barely run, and the can opener and the electric toothbrush that are broken. Appliances make me feel so dependent on them. They make me feel all the more passive.

Yesterday, I woke up, and I realized that it was twelve days before July 5, and I began to think to myself, "Maybe I should not have the baby." It seems so difficult, especially in this environment. Something in me wants to have another baby, and Frank has promised me a cleaning lady, a babysitter, and a typist, and he got a pool for the kids. He's tried to do so much. The trouble is that when I tell him something, or complain about something, he starts helping me. But yesterday, I was counting the days, and I was thinking, "Maybe, I should have an abortion because the physical drain is too much. I don't know."

Frank was going to unhook the sprinkler from the hose so that I could fill Katherine's tub, but when I went out there, the sprinkler was still connected. I thought, "Damn it," but I went ahead and got it disconnected, and then I turned on the water. No water was coming out. Then I realized that I had disconnected the sprinkler on the end of the hose, but this hose was an extension hose. Frank had disconnected the two hoses from each other. It annoyed me. He said that he was going to disconnect the sprinkler, and what he did was separate the two hoses. My anger is closer to the surface than ever before. The person I present to the outside world is more pleasant. We develop personas to present to others out there. I was wondering why it is that we don't have our pleasant, interesting personas at home. It would be different if you were with little children from nine to five. After a while, this round-the-clock vigilance wears on you; your patience is worn thin, or the children grind you down. What you're left with is raw personality. It's very, very hard to be sick and take care of little ones besides. There are probably a lot of things that I can tell myself; in any case, I just feel exhausted, depleted, and bored. My repertoire of activities is limited: carrying the laundry up and down the stairs and loading and unloading the dishwasher.

I really do think the children are fascinating. I think they are both masterpieces, fantastically smart and beautiful, and I wouldn't change them in any way. To watch Katherine's emerging personality is amazing. I wouldn't want to do anything else at this point except watch the children, but I think that if there were just one day a week that I did actually have off or if I had a little more time for myself, it would make a very big difference. Although I like things as they are, there is almost no way to meet my individual needs; after all, I do have some individual needs.

I have also had a strange sensation, like being attached to everything. The other day, I went into the bathroom to brush my teeth, and the electric toothbrush kept falling off the head or the motor. I wanted to say ouch when that happened. Just now, I put my hand on the yellow butterfly chair with the yellow canvas seat, and I noticed the top of it has a hole on one end. Everything I pick up or everything I touch now has a hole in it or a crack, and I have a feeling of being attached to it as if it's something personal. It's a little bit like sitting down to eat dinner when Katherine is in the high chair; it gives me butterflies in my stomach because I'm so afraid she's either going to throw her dish across the room or she's going to fall out of the high chair, and I'm in a state of tension, ready to grab the dish, the high chair, or her. There's always this feeling. It's tension, poised and waiting. I have to control this thing that might suddenly get out of order. I thought about our neighbor Earl's personality. He is probably very lively because he never had parents. I was thinking of him in contrast to Frank. Frank always says how much he likes processes, and it's true. To me, he takes processes to an almost frightening extent. He can get completely absorbed in it. He has very little drive to complete anything. Like that trip to Baltimore where he went with his father—how upset his father was because they were late. Frank kept telling him to enjoy the process. Earl is geared toward goals. Right down the line. I'm sure that it's because he lacked parents, and he felt that he had to be his own parent. I think I felt a little bit that way as a teenager. I would have welcomed someone to give me a little guidance. But I was caught up in the form and didn't really have a chance for the content. I was so into goals that I didn't put the same effort into existence. I think that does have something to do with parents.

I think it's strange too that if you're a woman and if you've been switched on to goals and then suddenly, you're in a position where you want to be involved with existence, sometimes, it's very frustrating. The only way you've known how to operate is to have goals, and if you don't have some little realm in which you can work toward a goal, it's very frustrating. I guess I'm wondering about all of this because of the statement that Margaret Mead made about kids being brought up and knowing nothing but the emotions of the modern suburban home—in other words, knowing only these emotions and being out of touch with the real world. What are the emotions in the modern suburban home? What are the emotions under the surface of this personality? And when you are switched on to goals or if you have a job—responsibility—it takes a certain amount of energy just to commute back and forth, to get there and function, so that all these emotions are constantly in a state of repression, in the service of getting things done. You operate with a kind of persona, I guess. So what are all these emotions? Do they come from the unconscious mind, the grotesque and infantile and fearful parts of the unconscious? Should they be repressed in the interest of navigating in the outside world, the world of adult business? The other thing that I wondered about is if anybody who is an artist and works at home has these feelings and just pours them into his work, probably, what he does is give form to these feelings. I wonder if his situation is something like the situation of housewives at home, except that writers or painters who live alone and just write or paint usually have a rip-roaring social life. They go to the café every single night. Or they live in a place like Greenwich Village. They live surrounded by people doing similar things, and so it isn't as though they never get away. What is the difference between that kind of life and, say, ours? You see somebody like the artist that I saw on TV, Hundertwasser. What they do is give form to what's inside them. These women at home . . . I think that when the mask that you have when you are with other adults and out in the world is taken off and you are home all the time with the kids, you find yourself roaming around in the jungle of your own unconscious mind. It seems to me that the answer is not to put the repressive lid on all of this. Maybe, it's better to take a look at what's there. Maybe, this is the next thing that's going to come into form. I'm convinced that's what the artist does. The only difference is that the artist has the technology and a certain consciousness of at least some aspects of this. This is his working material, his compost heap.

When I think of my own mother, I think of the difference, when I was about three, between being at my grandmother's and being at home with my mother. My grandmother always had my three unmarried uncles in and out and around, and they had friends with them. There was always a lot of laughter and joking and fantastic storytelling about what they'd done and what they'd seen and what people were doing. At the same time, all kinds of things were coming out of the oven to the table. These people seemed to me so happy. With my mother, all I had was feelings of sadness, so it was a relief to go to my grandmother's. These feelings were too much, that intensity all the time was too much. I remember being sick when I was eight years old; I had been crying for days with a pain on my side. I had been vomiting. Finally, my mother took me over to the Children's Hospital in Boston. I had never felt such an intense feeling of relief to get away from my mother because my mother was so worried about me I couldn't stand it. Whereas once I got into the hands of the nurses and the doctors, they had a more cheery, matter-of-fact attitude; they were kind and friendly. It was like the sun coming out and all the clouds lifting off and the terrible pressure passing. In a way, I can see that pressure like that might lead to drugs or to street people when children are only with this kind of oppressed emotion. It is so contagious and strong that it's frightening. The mother herself can't get away from it, so how can the children? You're trapped together in these feelings, so a child would never want to be in the house. You would never willingly give yourself a chance to deal with these inner feelings. You probably wouldn't have a house of your own. The ideal life is that everybody has a home, but I do think that it probably would be normal to live in a hotel or to have a studio with a couch in it. It doesn't have to be a place like a living room, but it's got to be a place where you can do something, where you have a chance to act out your inner drama a little bit. If you never have a home, you'd never go through the birth of the self. If you always want to be in an impersonal setting, it is like not creating anything yourself or giving form to anything or to yourself. You have to get your hands into something.

I can see why young people would want to get away from anything resembling being at home, if they do have an unhappy suburban mother, but they never develop any kind of peace within themselves. They are at war with themselves. Maybe, that's why so many go to drugs. They find an escape from home and then later from the constant stimulation of the street.

When I look back at my own education that, I think, I created somewhat on my job but almost everything that I dealt with was what other people had given me, and I digested it, and I regurgitated it. I don't know what it means in terms of women who stay at home and how they are doing things differently from the artist. Truly, the right thing can't be to always live with a lid on yourself, always live as though you are a nurse in a hospital or a dentist or a librarian where time is spent getting ready to go to work, then going to work, working, dealing with the community at work and the people you just run into. You don't have to arrange to meet them. You just bump into them. You see other people. This is one world. But there's also the other, the subjective world. What the artist does is make the subjective world objective. In a way, the subjective world is "in" and the objective world is "out." The artist has been to art school or has studied a craft and has a technology. He's been in both worlds. He's in, then out, then back in. Maybe, this is what women are going to have to do in order to give some kind of form to the seething chaos that they are.

The more I think about Margaret Mead's review of Elizabeth Janeway's book, the more I realize there's a slight implication that the world out there, the man's world, the objective world, the world of the street and the city, is more real than, say, the world of the isolated subjective individual. The big difference between a woman at home and a woman with a job is that what is underneath the personality of the woman at work is more greatly repressed. The material that comes up when a mother is home all the time is very real. Women at home with small children usually work very hard. It's an emotional job, and her own training, especially if she's gone through college or done graduate work, could be a handicap. It's amazing how much time and effort goes into your professional life and your ego life: your clothes and your appointments and the things you do out in the world. The only people that are an exception to this are artists because they are putting their guts on paper. They have to spend a lot of time alone, and they work in a personal environment, so they would probably be the exception. But all the women that are lawyers, doctors, librarians, judges, school teachers, or secretaries—it's not only that they retrained for the possibilities of "out" and all their skills and the tremendous amount of time and effort and energy they put into these things, but that these things are also really surface, and when you are at home with small children, it's not as though you can get up in the morning and take your shower, select what you are going to wear that day, get dressed, and appear on the job at a certain time. Now would you have lunch with your colleagues and then finish at a certain time, having a certain number of hours to yourself. I really am impressed by any mother who takes care of her house herself, and has small children, gets the children breakfast, lunch, and dinner, gives them a bath every day, puts them in for a nap, and then, if she can, spends some time in the evening reading them a story or playing with them during the day; I think that is fantastic. She also does other things in the house too. I think that what happens is she is suddenly so busy taking care of one, two, or three children she doesn't really have any more time for her ego life. Something else happens to women, and I would really like to know what it is. Their ego disappears. Or their ego disappears, and they sink into their own unconscious; the veneer of the civilized self vanishes, and it's partly because they work so hard and don't even have time to give themselves the attention to make themselves feel civilized. It is surface ego that goes. This ego—similar to one-tenth of the iceberg above the surface—is gone because it has no function in this kind of life. What you are left with is the seething mass of life, the chaotic mass churning just beneath civility, like a tub of guts, primal. We are brought up so that there is no development from inside of us to the outside. Life should develop from the inside out, but it doesn't with the extrinsic education we have. Our development is greasepaint: it's just slapped on to the outside, and most of it doesn't get integrated, and the deepest levels of the personality are neglected. No wonder under the thin surface, people are primitive. With mothers at home full-time, it's the same. The ego completely vanishes.

The ego of my mother's sister Theresa, or Connie's sister Tina, is like a thin little gossamer that just crumbles. I think of the story of Immanuel Rath, the schoolmaster in the film *The Blue Angel*, everything about his personality is external, and once he goes internal, he disintegrates. He's formless. I think that with people that are integrated or have artistic personalities—people that are in touch with their deepest selves—ego disintegration is much less likely to occur. I would guess that Emily or, maybe, Connie Stark could live the life of a woman with two or three small children and not really be the same as the mother in the modern suburban home whose children go to drugs because the child is familiar only with the emotions of the modern suburban home. These people have probably felt their emotions before. But I think that for most people, because their education is so external, ego disintegration would be inevitable if they were suddenly thrust upon themselves, isolated in the suburbs with only children to talk to. Connie's sister is a good example of someone who becomes almost grotesquely brutal. I've seen other women go through a transformation after they get married and have a baby. I've often wondered why. There was a woman who lived across the street from my friend Jimmy McLaughlin. We always called her Mickey's mother because she was married and the strange thing is that I remembered her before Mickey was born. She had been an attractive blond. She had one child, and after the child got to be about two, she would sit out on the front step during most of the day watching him, and all she did was call to him, "Mickey, Mickey, Mickey." She'd be croaking at him. She used to sit and smoke and throw cigarette butts in the street. She got more and more slovenly looking. Each time that I saw her, she looked worse. Then she would be sitting with a can of beer screaming at her child. Her hair got more greasy-looking; it hung down and clung to her neck. She looked as though she wore no underwear under her dresses, and her dresses were unkempt. She used to sit there, smoke, drink beer, and bark at her child. Sometimes, I'd see her husband sitting there, and in the evenings, they would fight. Then she began to develop a hacking cough. Then she lost all of her teeth. Then she became pregnant and had another baby. I don't know what happened to her after that, but in a period of maybe two years, it was incredible to see such a striking woman simply disintegrate. I suppose there might have been something wrong with her health, but I've seen this so much in a less extreme form. It happens so often, and I can only think that the person was never in touch with one's own inner self, undeveloped as that self may be. She has veneer, a veneer of a civilized ego, and in a situation where that ego is not encouraged or supported but is isolated, it loses its reason for existing.

It's like brainwashing where there is no ego gratification. The person can be broken right down. If a woman is dependant on her husband for ego gratification, she'll lose her reason for existing too because chances are, there will be very little support forthcoming. Once this goes, what's left is a kind of primitive person. I wonder if the same thing would happen to men who stayed home. I wonder if they are so far away from their inner selves that there isn't even an inner self to make contact with. Many old people who stay isolated regress. One could say, "Go out and get a job and be in touch with the rest of the world." It covers up the symptoms. If women are closer to nature than men, then there's a great deal of nature there that's going to require looking at, becoming conscious of, and dealing with. It's surprising, in a way, that a woman can have nurses training, for example, and have worked a couple years and then be at home with small children. She's in about the same shape as the high school graduate.

I think there is little connection between a woman's ego and her instinct. Connie's mother is another example of that. She had such a strong desire to marry and have children. With some women, the desire is so strong that they're willing to destroy their mind in order to do it. It shows the extent to which women will go to procreate. The desire is stronger than ego drives or other drives, but I think that there'll be a whole new section of the iceberg brought up pretty soon. There'll be two-tenths of the iceberg brought up for inspection, and it won't be just the one-tenth that's visible. I wonder if women are going to have to go through this "doing." They'll all have to be trained for "out." Until they realize that there is something wrong with that or it is not deeply fulfilling enough or that there are certain things in a woman's nature that aren't sufficiently satisfied by it, they'll have to first go "out" to discover it, all over again, but it will really be completely different. I had to go "out" first before I could see any possibility of "in." But these women who are "in" all the time are probably in a bad way, and so are the ones who have had a little bit of training for "out" but never go as far in it as they want to go. These other urges that are unconscious take hold, and they always think of "out" as the zenith of their lives. It's a shame that many women get so little out of their children. They not only learn nothing from them, but they get so little out of the whole experience. I would like to get as much out of it as I could and explore all the possibilities of "in." I don't know whether I can.

Sometimes, I feel so frustrated, losing patience, but I guess it's something I have to work at. I guess that's why I want to have a third baby. I want to have another chance to make it perfect, and all these emotions that I have, I don't want them to harm the children. In a way, I don't think that the way to greater growth for me is to go back and get my old job back at the Library of Congress. The emotions that I feel would be swept under the rug and stay there. I think that for my own development, I have to explore these feelings. I don't want to harm the children by doing it, but it's a chance to become more conscious. It's going to be hard to do, and I suspect I haven't done very well so far.

I guess if I were in a fabulous and stimulating atmosphere, I would just tend to be stimulated and be stimulated and be stimulated, and I would never really go inward and explore my experiences in life. I don't mind not going to galleries and bookstores so much myself, but I do wish there were more places to take the children to besides the backyard.

Monday, July 26, 1971

It's been a fantastically long time since I've recorded in this pregnancy diary. There were two reasons why I haven't recorded anything before now. One of them is that we have started the children in swimming lessons, and the swimming lessons started on July 5. We completed two weeks of lessons and then decided to enroll the children again and go for two more weeks. This means setting the alarm and getting up at about 7:00 a.m. and getting back here for lunch about noontime; we stop at the store or do an errand on the way home. That has taken quite a big chunk of time out of the day. The other reason is that Mrs. Fisk, who has been typing the motherhood tapes, brought back four pages the first week. She also gave me the machine, so I listened to the fourteen pages and then gave it to her for corrections. Then she brought me seventeen pages, and I've gone through that. So whatever free time I have had in the afternoon when the children had been napping, I used to revise the typed manuscript. It takes quite a long time to listen to the tape and compare it to the typed version.

From the time that I last recorded, I felt not only tired, but bored, which is really unusual for me. I felt bored and empty, and even the view from my living room window didn't interest me as much as it usually does. That was the thing I noticed most strongly, and it surprised me. Usually, I could look out the window at the scene and be invigorated because it's so beautiful across the way. But it was so hot that there wasn't even a breeze to move the leaves on the trees. It was like looking at a picture. It wasn't like looking at the ocean or a fire or something that's moving. It was absolutely still.

I would take the children out, but it was absolutely excruciating for me to stand. I would go up to the swings with Katherine, but just standing up there in the hot, hot sun seemed so difficult. The combination of the heat and the standing was too much.

There were a couple of afternoons when the children would wake up at 4:00 p.m., and I would ask myself, "How am I going to go on?" It's like working from seven to three and from three to eleven. It's like working two eight-hour shifts. Wednesday, when Frank was here, I felt so depressed and tired that all of a sudden, I couldn't go on, and I just cried and cried and cried. I couldn't help it. I felt that I didn't have the strength. To some extent, up until July 5, when the matter was closed, I did wonder whether I should have an abortion. The thing is that between the time that Katherine was born and now, I never really resolved in my own mind whether I wanted to have a third baby or not. And somewhere, down in my deepest layers or levels, I would like to have one more, but the work—just taking care of Thomas and Katherine seems so, so hard. One day, I was up at the swings, and the mailman came and brought a letter from Mrs. Ulanoff. I had written to her on Anna's suggestion, asking her if she knew of anything on motherhood. I got a letter from her, and she said that Helene Deutsch's book on motherhood, which is volume two of her classic work on the psychology of women, is the best-known work on the subject of motherhood. The reply came from Mrs. Ulanoff, and then I saw the first autumn leaf. I noticed that there was a yellow leaf on the ground, and my heart leapt for joy. It leapt for joy because I absolutely love the autumn. I love the autumn in New England, but I love the autumn here even more. It lasts longer. Thank goodness for air-conditioning. It is so hot here that when you are in an air-conditioned place for a while and you go outside, you can hardly relate to the outside. In the fantastic heat, it seems as though everything is dead, nothing moves. It is as though there is a fantastic weight on my head. The summers in New England were much more pleasant than summers here. I don't care that much for the summers here. When I saw the autumn leaf, it was a turning point. I told myself autumn is coming and, that in itself made me feel happy. Autumn is a time of fantastic expectation. It seems like the whole world is pregnant. The feelings that people associate with spring I associate with autumn. Maybe, it's harvest, but from my birthday to Christmas or New Year, that's the half of the year that I prefer. I suddenly began to feel very happy again. I had been bereft of all of my inner resources. I'm sure that it was the pregnancy, the fact that I wasn't getting the high or a marvelous feeling from being pregnant yet is because I wasn't far enough along into the pregnancy. It was the early stages, and my body wasn't producing its regular hormones. It was like being neither here nor there. At any rate, I suddenly did feel much better. I am very happy about being pregnant. I think that in some ways, I am rather old at age thirty-nine. I don't have as much energy, and I do have other interests in life, but still, we do have two such beautiful children. It's as though I want to extend this period a little longer. I am happy about it. I think that I would feel that this time is really enough. This is like having two desserts. I could probably get by with one, I might be longing for another, but this will take care of that longing. I will have had enough of babies and diapers. There will be no doubt in my mind that this is it. Seeing that autumn leaf ended a barren period.

The National Gallery calendar of events for July came in the mail, and I saw a description of a series of talks on ten cities that, at certain times in history, have been centers for great artistic development. That sounds fantastic, and I told Frank, "Wouldn't it be nice to see this?" On the Fourth of July, we went to a lecture at the National Gallery, and Frank's parents watched the children. It really was not as interesting as I thought that subject could have been. There was a lot of details about altar pieces. I didn't think it was that good because it read like a description of the slides rather than some of the reasons why Sienna in the fourteenth century should produce whatever it produced. There were a few slides of present-day Sienna pageants shown, where the buildings are the same buildings that were standing in the fourteenth century. That was interesting to see. We didn't go back to any of the other lectures, but it was fun to go to that one.

I started thinking about what I am going to do—it's very strange, like being in high school and thinking of what I am going to do with my life. Something like that. I feel incredibly young as though I have been born again, born anew. I'm more and more myself, more and more pre-Thomas, so to speak. The world seems a terribly exciting place and a terribly interesting place.

I wanted to have a child, and at least three years have gone by. I had the desire growing in me, and now, it is beginning to bear fruit. I'm wondering about what I'm going to do even though I know what life will probably be like for the next two years. That's how I can tell I'm finishing up with the pregnancy and baby cycle. I think about women like Dr. Warner, who works in Dr. Molning's office. She seems like a very nice person, an interesting woman. She apparently doesn't feel that she has to live in the city. She's out in an area like this, and she's contributing something to it, so to speak. Her youngest child is seven months old. Or I think of Lesley Branck. She got married and had a baby who would be about two years old now, and then she had a second one about nine months ago. Although her two-year-old baby died, she has not stopped working at the library. Then I think of Mrs. Ulanoff, who had one baby, and may or may not have more children. She's a Jungian analyst and also a theologian. I think of women like them, and I wonder what I am going to do. Every now and then, Frank says, "Wouldn't it be a good idea for you to get a job?" I could get a job in one of the school libraries here. I could be home when the children were home, and I could have my summers free. I have always bristled, for all kinds of reasons, when he says that. In the first place, I want to be the one to decide. In the second place, he never wants to do extra work, yet he's always thinking up jobs for me, and my response is "When you are thinking about jobs, why don't you think of one for yourself? Think of yourself, Frank, or else start an employment agency." One particular morning, we had been driving through the Patuxent Wild Life Refuge, and we passed several buildings there, and Frank asked why I would not want to work there. I said maybe I would if it had been the Air and Space Museum Library. I think that would be so exciting. It would be fabulous. It's got to be more than just a job. I feel I have to compensate for living here. But more than that, I want to do other things. I had thought somewhat about becoming a Jungian analyst. I keep telling Anna that I think she should become a Jungian analyst. I didn't know that you could become a Jungian analyst without going to medical school. Sometimes, I think that would be fascinating. I wrote to the Jung Foundation in New York and was sent a catalog of their program for training. I was wondering if it would be possible to become an analyst. First, you need a hundred hours of analysis. There is a woman listed as being a Jungian analyst in the Maryland suburban phone book, but she is listed with just an address. It doesn't say where her office is or when office hours are. She's in Chevy Chase or Bethesda. I thought vaguely about getting in touch with her, but there were a lot of things that I wanted to read first. I want to study some more and read Kate Millet and Germaine Greer and the books that I have in my father's bookcase. I also want very much to write. I'd like to work in a library dedicated to women in art or about women artists or women writers or in a library on women.

Over the Fourth of July weekend on Sunday, it was hot, and we had the air-conditioning on and all the blinds down, and we cooked steak. It wasn't special or anything. Steak and salad. Frank and I had dinner at the dining table. The children were sleeping. It is so hard to eat with Katherine Louise. She throws her food, and I'm always trying to grab her, thinking she's going to fall right out of her high chair. Most of the time, meals are stressful. This time, the children were sleeping, and it was the most glorious experience. We had new Merrimeko place mats, which I just love because they are green. It was so pleasant to sit down with Frank. We talked, and I had asked him earlier if he wanted to go down to the gallery to hear a lecture on Venice or Florence. He said he felt that he had too many things to do, so I thought, "Well, it is nicer to be able to create an atmosphere and to create an environment where you feel that you don't have to go out to a restaurant or someplace special to get the sensation of being in love. It means more to me to be able to do that than to go to a gallery. But somehow, suddenly, the combination of lectures at the gallery and the letter from Mrs. Ulanoff made me think that just to see the kind of things that are listed under "motherhood" in the Jung Foundation Library would be exciting.

Just watching the children is more than a full-time job. To give them anything at all, I feel that I need some time to myself and need help with the house. Frank was extremely nice and kind. He said that when the baby is born, I should probably have a nurse at home from the hospital to help me with the baby. And he said that I could get a cleaning woman and more babysitting help. He really couldn't possibly do much more than that as far as offering me help. So I started to call all the agencies that I could. Naturally, I got a lot of what you might call bum steers, so I spent time and time and time and time on the phone. I was told they would call back. At the agency that seemed the most promising, Milford, the woman filled out applications and asked me questions about the person's duties and how much the person would have to be paid, what the fee was, and she said she thought she could probably find someone from this area who had a car. It was a Mrs. Smith at Milford that I had talked to, and calling her back, I was given a run around about how the office was moving over their Fourth of July weekend. A couple of times, I was told that Mrs. Smith was unavailable because she was visiting the new office. Finally, I was told that Milford had discontinued its daytime domestic help. They were only dealing now with live-ins. So I said I'd like to inquire about a live-in, and I found this interesting because I was told the women were all from the Caribbean and South or Central America, with something like a year guarantee, and they got $60 a week for a five-day week. You could either have one that's young, like twenty, or one that's settled and middle-aged like fifty. I was told the things they do. It would be impossible to put anybody up here. The place is much too small, for one thing, and it would only be possible if I were working. Anyway, I thought that was interesting. Compare them with the women who can get somebody like that to come in; the difference in the work some women have to do and what others have to do is unbelievable. Women who can afford to have somebody like that come and live in their homes have someone to do all the time-consuming hard work. In my own case, I feel that would be justified only if I were professionally employed.

I had just about given up trying to find household help. The agencies in Washington seem to handle mostly black women who come out on a daily basis from Southeast Washington. But there isn't any bus service out here, so that's out of the question. One of the things that upset me was the thought that I can't even afford to live in a place like this because there are absolutely no services. How will it ever be possible to even think of doing anything like taking on a job or spending more time writing or doing anything at all like that when one can't even get a babysitter? You can't get anybody. It's really hopeless. In addition to that, I began to think that I would try to get a babysitter to look after Katherine in the afternoon for two hours, from four to six, maybe four days a week. I called Joan Sutter, who said she would come over. I thought that during the summer, I would try to use Mandy Parkland as a sitter although I have to go over there and pick her up, but it turns out Mandy is pregnant. She's going to have a baby around the first part of September, so I can't ask her because it would be hard for her to run around after Katherine. More than that, though, is the problem of having to drive over there and get her. It's more than I can do. Joan said she would come over, and she did. Katherine just screamed and screamed. After a week or so, we're sitting out there with them and trying to distract Katherine Louise and get Thomas there and the Lister kids were over. I was standing on my head trying to think of things that I could do to keep her amused and get her involved in something before I disappeared, before she realized I was gone. No sooner did I succeed in getting Katherine to stay out with Joan for ten minutes when Joan called and said she had to go to Pennsylvania. No cleaning lady, no babysitter. That's really not so good, but Beth, who lives next door, came. Katherine Louise was pretty much the same with Beth. Joan is now back, and by a fluke, it turned out that a patient happened to stop by to tell Frank about a cleaning lady who has a car pool. It seems that there is a car pool of cleaning ladies who go to Cheverly, and this Cheverly patient happens to have a sister-in-law who lives in Kettering. So the cleaning lady comes to Kettering. Frank gave this woman our number, and I thought she probably wouldn't call, so I started looking up everybody by the name of Zoens in the phone book, trying to find this Jeanette Zoens to ask her how I could get in touch with her cleaning lady. Anyway, I didn't have to do that. The cleaning lady, Mrs. Adams, called here, and so if all works out the way it's planned, she's supposed to come here every other Monday. I felt happy, fantastically happy, because that will make such a big difference to me. Once I started doing the motherhood recording around the first part of February, I decided I'd give the first couple of hours of every day to housework—dishes, laundry, and vacuuming—because I've got to make some time for myself. I was pleased about it all, and then Joan came back again. I'm still working with her. I had managed to persuade Frank to let me get a Sony tape recorder because I wanted to get my motherhood tapes typed. But the thought of having a typist sitting in the living room while I'm trying to watch my children seemed absolutely mad. Mrs. Fisk said she wouldn't do the typing unless she could do it at home. I began to see all the possibilities of having a portable Sony tape recorder because I could take the tape recorder with me anywhere as long as there was an electric outlet. I could control it more than the Tanberg. Also, one could type from it more easily. There were all kinds of ramifications I could see. I had persuaded Frank to get it for me, and I thought I had a typist all lined up. She was going to charge $1.75 a page for single-spaced typing. From calling around to different places, investigating, besides calling all around about a cleaning lady, I've also been calling all around about a typist or transcriber. It seems to me that Mrs. Fisk is quite cheap, and she's nearby. It was all set up. I had given her the equivalent of about a third of the motherhood tapes. It just so happened that it was on my birthday that she telephoned me. She had the tape for maybe three or four days. After the cleaning lady fell through, and it looked like Joan fell through, and Mandy got pregnant, she called and said, "Do you realize how much this is going to cost? I have typed one side of one cassette, and it's equivalent to ten single-spaced pages." The total job would cost $840. Needless to say, I had a shock right there, so I called her back and said, "Let me talk to my husband about it." I was figuring in terms of $200 for this one thing; I thought Frank would faint at $200. When I realized that was only one-quarter of it and it would be $840, I was somewhat taken aback by that price. So I called her back and asked her to give me a little more time to think it over. So I thought about it. Frank kept saying, "There's this typewriter in my office." Frank wanted to type it. Then he said that maybe, Denise, his office assistant, could type it, or Mandy Parkland's sister or a student at the University of Maryland. I called Denise, and she couldn't do it and didn't know anyone who could. I called Mandy Parkland's sister Sharon. She never called back. I called the University of Maryland, and they don't list jobs in their placement office that are in homes or just for individuals. I called some transcribing places downtown, and to have it officially transcribed would be even more expensive than having Mrs. Fisk, and these places all said things like "and it's a rough draft too." Listening to the first section, I think Mrs. Fisk is doing an excellent job. If I had any of these other services do it, I don't think they would do even as good a job as she is doing. I do think it's an expensive service, but I don't think she's overcharging. That seemed like the blow to end all blows—$840! Then I thought about having my mother type it. I don't like to ask her. I'd rather give it to somebody who's impersonal because I don't know what I've said. But at $840, you might think twice. Besides, I'd have to send the tape machine up to my mother, and I would need a lot more cassettes. I couldn't have the typing back and forth and back and forth, as I can with Mrs. Fisk. I decided that the best thing to do would be to let her type $200 worth of manuscript. Two hundred dollars would be a lot, that would be about 120 pages. At least, I could see what it looked like, and I could let somebody else read it. Then I could decide whether it would be worth it to try to have my mother type it. I had to persuade Frank to do that. Finally, he was agreeable, and I felt quite pleased about that, having at least worked it out to that small extent.

Anna called me on my birthday, July 10, to wish me a happy birthday. It was so great to talk to her. I told her about my motherhood tapes, and she asked me if she could read it. Maybe, I will let her read it. It was on the thirteenth that Mrs. Fisk called and said how much it was going to be, and I thought, "If I don't get any of it typed, no one can read it." I was very happy to be able to start getting some of it typed. I have seen what Mrs. Fisk has done, and I'm really very pleased with the typing. It was interesting to talk to Anna because she said that Jung said the basic principle of the unconscious is the eternal feminine. She also said that she thought it was really interesting that all at the same time, there was an awareness of the rape of nature and the subjugation of women and the brutality to man's own inner life. On the Fourth of July, we had gone on a picnic. Our neighbors, the Tates and the Plows, had an impromptu picnic. Everybody in the neighborhood came and brought his own meat, and it was fun. Sylvia gave me whiskey sours. It was backyardsville, but still, it was pleasant to talk to everybody. I began to feel that Kettering is a wasteland in the desert. I began to think about cities and how great cities are. I have to invent a mythology for why I'm not in a city. I have to overcompensate. I have to create my own Kepes. I have to wean myself. Go to the headwaters of the Orinoco or the Bramaputra rivers. What better place to do it than here? Maybe, there is something to be gained from being here. Jeannette, my next-door neighbor, sent me a card and said she hoped it would be my best birthday ever. I have decided that it is my best birthday. It is absolutely my best birthday, and I think that's really something to be able to say that. My thirty-ninth birthday.

Wednesday, August 4, 1971

I feel so busy and rushed as though I'm running, running, running, just to get a couple of minutes to myself. It's like the carrot that's held just out of my reach. I never get the carrot. When I got married, I thought I was going to escape certain of my own imprisonments, and then after Thomas was born, it seemed that I had a whole new set of imprisonments. Gradually, though, I think I've worked my way through those, and now, it's just a question of time.

Yesterday, Katherine Louise took no nap at all, and not only did she have no nap, but at ten-thirty last night, she was still awake. Finally, I asked Frank if he'd watch her for me for a little while; I told him, if she wasn't asleep in an hour, to wake me up, and I'd watch her. So he got her up and read to her, and then she went to bed, I guess, at eleven-thirty. The day before, she took a nap for maybe an hour. By the time I put her in for her nap, Frank went to work, and I pried Thomas away from Freddy and Gregory, she was awake.

On Sunday, the Dicksons came for dinner. The day was pleasant, but still, it was rush, rush, rush. I got up in the morning and made an angel food cake. I put the batter in the pan the wrong way, so I had to empty it, reassemble the pan, put the batter back in, and then after it was cool, frost it. Then I had to take a shower with Katherine, get breakfast, clean up after breakfast, clean the house a little, take the children out, get lunch, put the children in for their naps, set the table up for the dinner, and cook the dinner. It's just go, go, go.

Saturday, the day before that, I had Mandy Parkland come over, and I went downtown and got my haircut. It was pleasant. I was very happy to go downtown and have a little time to myself. When I came back, I had the feeling that Frank was far away from me. I came back and gave Mandy a ride home, with Katherine Louise in the car. Thomas was still asleep. When I came back, Thomas was still asleep, and Frank was painting the tires on the Volkswagen. He had the car all jacked up, which meant that if one of the kids leaned against it, it could fall over on them. I brought Katherine in the house. Finally, Thomas got up, but it was raining out, and the Lister kids came in, and they were roughhousing. I made pizza for dinner, and neither one of the children ate a bit of it. That night, both children were awake from two to four in the morning. First, one would cry; then, the other would cry. Katherine was coughing more. I go downtown and get a few hours of what Hortense Calisher would call "playing single" (though I don't really think of it that way), and then when I come back, things are in much more of a mess than if I hadn't left. The children seem to me to reflect my absence. They act more fussy, and they don't want to go to sleep. Maybe, I imagined it. Maybe, they would have been awake from two to four in the morning anyway. But it's very strange. The last hour or so when I'm out, I get frantic to come back, really frantic. I begin to imagine that all kinds of horrible things have happened. Something steps up my pace, anxiety steps it up, and my thoughts begin to dart around more, and although I try to think of something else, my thoughts get pulled right back on the track of the children. I keep imagining that something had happened to Katherine Louise. So going away like that does have its price. I do keep telling myself that it is necessary to get out and get away every once in a while. I do have to get my haircut once in a while and go to the doctor.

I can't quite remember as far back as Friday, but it has been days and days and days since I have gotten any time to myself. I have wanted to record in my diary something about the pregnancy and do some of the corrections on the motherhood manuscript. I don't know whether I should do any corrections on it now or just wait until I get the tape recorder back and then do it all then. It's surprising how much time it takes to do the corrections.

I have the cleaning lady, and I do have Joan to come over, and I can get Mandy Parkland to come over on a Saturday so that I can do more things and have a little more time. But the cleaning lady didn't show up on Monday, and Katherine is not happy with Joan. Joan takes her out, in again, out again, and in some ways, it's more of a strain to have her around. I can't settle down to actually record, and I can't read because they're in and out, in and out. Katherine seems to be getting gradually—but only very, very gradually—more used to Joan. Each weekend time is lost. We have to start all over again on Monday.

My feelings about the motherhood project, seeing it typed, are very strange. It was only about Friday before I had a chance to read it, but on Wednesday night, I had started to read the first two pages, and I was disappointed. It seemed to me so boring. All this business about drinking sixteen glasses of water a day and washing my nipples before and after breast feeding and boiling the water seemed just plain boring. Maybe, it was for that reason that I didn't have time to reedit for a couple of days. Frank read it before I did. It was sitting on the red desk, so he picked it up, and I felt strange when he was reading it because I hadn't read it, and I wondered if I'd said anything about Frank that would upset him. He was reading it, and I was wondering what his reaction would be. He said to me, "Um, well, maybe, sometime, I'll really know you." And he said, "I didn't know you didn't like Cherry Hill that much." And he said, "I didn't know that Martin Luther King's death upset you that much." He then said to me, "Maybe, sometime, what you should do is turn on the tape recorder and free-associate." He said that he thought the beginning started a little slow because of getting used to doing the recording, but he said, "Once you get going, it's really very interesting." When I did read it, I thought the pace did pick up, and it did get a little more interesting as it went along.

There is the question of what to do when Mrs. Fisk finishes this much. She's got twelve hours, which is somewhere between a fourth and a third of the tape, and it's going to be something like 120 pages. The question is what to do with the rest of it. It is very expensive to have her type it. I don't know if I could ask my mother. It seems too personal, though I didn't talk about sex. There is a whole new thing that I feel myself reacting to. I alternate between disappointment and pleasure. I don't know if I should show it to anybody else. I don't know what I'm going to do with it. Just having the corrections made seems like a big thing, and I do want to do this pregnancy diary and keep it up for a while after the baby is born. There are other things that I want to do too. The other things are vague in my mind.

I just put Katherine Louise into her crib with a bottle. She's talking in there and drinking her bottle. I have to slightly cheat a little on the kids. I only do this when they are sleeping, but like now, Katherine's not exactly sleeping. But I didn't start this until Thomas was three years old and Katherine was a year and a half, so I really didn't feel too bad about that.

I am very glad that I feel as well as I do. I think I'm over the hump of the first three months, the tiredness and the worry over the possibility of a miscarriage. I feel a lot better, and it is a joy to be able to do this recording. I don't think I could ever write down that much. It's an entirely different process. And the result, of course, seems very different.

I'm reading *Up the Sandbox* right now by Ann Richardson Roife. It is so cleverly written. She has done such a good job. There are parts of it that remind me a little bit of Katherine Mansfield—for example, when she's describing a rather elderly couple in the park, the lady having perfectly curled and tinted hair and the man stopping by in the bakery every night and buying himself a little almond cake. But some of Katherine Mansfield's characters also seem pathetic, like retired lonely people who stop by in a bakery to buy a little cake for themselves. There are also times when her writing reminds me very much of Sylvia Plath. There is an undertow running through it, a concern with death. There are references to death and dying, experiences of wanting to shut death out. I haven't finished the book. I don't quite know what I think of it. I gave the review of *Up the Sandbox* in the *New York Times* to the Reals. I wish I still had it because the last sentence was disturbing; it was something like *The Sandbox* makes a point that feminist literature does not concede to but didn't go on to explain what it was. It did quote the heroine of the book saying something like, "There is one thing that I can do, and that is create another life. I can't build a bridge or do a piece of sculpture to go in a museum." I saw Emily about this time, and I asked her what she thought it meant. She said it meant that after you get your masters degree and after you get all fired up by Women's Liberation, you can't really do anything about the problems of inequality. I don't know whether that's true or not. Anyway, there are parts of the book that are very clever. The description of her feelings for her little daughter, Elizabeth, and also that of her relationship with her mother are touching. Then I think about what I have said, and I think, "Yuck!" But I keep thinking about what I've created. I still have to figure out what I want to do about getting the rest of that typed.

When I go for about four days and I don't have any time to myself, either in the evening or in the afternoon when the children are napping, I get very scattered. I haven't seen Jeannette Real since she got back from her vacation, and I feel a little guilty about it as though I am not friendly. She called me Tuesday to say that Kurt was sick and wasn't going to go to playschool with Thomas. I said, "We'll have to get together and have some coffee." I was going to call her this morning, but then with the prospect of having this little bit of time to myself after so long, I thought, "My God, that half an hour is just too precious." I just cannot share it with anybody. And so here I am, alone with this half an hour, glad that I'm not bleeding and not flat on my back. I do feel well, and it's good that I'll be able to work out something better with the cleaning lady and the babysitter. I usually feel great in the morning lately. As the day wears on, of course, I feel more droopy.

My mother called. It sounds as though she had a wonderful trip. She sounded great. She sent Frank and me two hand-knit sweaters from Ireland, and I just love mine. This Sunday, we are going to a champagne party for Claire Smith and Jim Roberts. They are supposed to be getting married today in Iowa, and next weekend, my sister, Louise, and her son, Gary, are coming here. Those are really nice things to look forward to. It makes a big difference to have something to look forward to. They are like peaks, and if I can keep jumping from peak to peak rather than getting stuck in the valleys, that's great.

I think I have overcome my problem about living in a development. I still feel, intellectually, the same way about developments as a way of life. When we say that humankind has to change its lifestyle if we are to survive on this planet, I think it is this particular lifestyle that's going to have to change, more than anything else. There is just so little to offer the kids. In a review of Elizabeth Janeway's *Man's World, Woman's Place* in the *New York Times*, Margaret Meade said that so many kids are turning to drugs because all they know is the emotions of the suburban home. I think there is something pathological about this way of life, but I personally think that I can survive it. I sometimes wonder what the price is. I wonder what it would have been like if I had married somebody in Boston, had continued working at the Rotch Library, and had two children. I keep telling myself that because of the experiences I have had, there must be some creative use to which I can put this experience. There must be some gain to be made out of the pain, something to be gleaned from it.

We have finished the four weeks of swimming lessons at the Y with the kids. It was exciting to get up in the morning and go somewhere, especially in the summer when the mornings are so beautiful. When we came back, both kids were so exhausted they took long naps. It's a little harder to watch Katherine around here, and it's probably a little more boring, although less tiring. One day, we drove to get gas, so we went in the other direction, and we passed Sil's dental office. He has a very impressive office on Colesville Road, what you might expect an affluent dentist to have. It's a brick house that is fairly close to the street. There is a little greenery in front of it, red brick with white trim, and an extremely well-manicured lawn. It's on a very busy thoroughfare, and there are lots of doctors' offices on either side of him.

Today is Claire's wedding, and Frank and I have been talking about that. She is marrying a man who is in charge of the Washington office of Standard Oil. I would guess that probably, he is wealthy. She is going to be moving back here, living in Potomac. But Sil's office was very impressive, and Frank thought that Sil was in such financial trouble that he couldn't afford Kettering and that this was a downhill step, but I don't think that was the case. I think that he was trying to move to a much more affluent neighborhood.

Frank and I have been talking about how important it is for Claire to have money. With us having two little children and another child on the way, I think, probably, we can't afford a family. Sometimes, it seems as if we are so poor. All our appliances are breaking down, and Frank does his own car repair, irons his own dental coats, and cuts his own hair. He claims he does all those things out of preference, but our car gets worse and worse looking each time, and our clothes get shabbier and shabbier. It is a strange sensation to realize what money does. I have always felt that in my whole life, before marriage, I always did what I wanted to do and was never hampered by the lack of money. When I listen to Frank, it seems as though all his life, he's been aware of money. He went to the University of Maryland. Joe Rydings was there. Maybe, it was Joe Rydings's grandfather, but he was a multimillionaire, and Frank was always aware that guys with money dated certain girls. It's very strange. I never was aware of privilege or class. I remember at Simmons, somebody pointed out Taylor Caldwell's daughter. She seemed so pathetic, like a kid who had spent her whole life at summer camp. But I am beginning to see what is meant by the American way of life and what money can do. In some ways, it's the first time as an adult I'm seeing what the lives of ordinary people are like, and I guess that I have aspirations, but they are not money aspirations. Sometimes, I wonder if having a cleaning lady would make me do anything any differently or would make me do more. I don't want to feel that my life is different from what it would be if I had money. I want to do what I want to do regardless of money. I keep telling myself that it hasn't made any difference. I think the only time that it has made any difference was after Thomas was born. I wish I had somebody I could have called to help me do things. I would have been happier, and maybe, I would have started writing. What I want to do more than anything else is write. Money probably wouldn't make that much difference in what I turned out. It would buy me time. I guess it depends on how much I can do the way things are, whether I can pay to have a typist, for example. But maybe, it's just an illusion. I refuse to believe that my life would be any different. Yet there are times when I ask myself, "What would my life be like if I had married somebody in Boston and continued my job there?" Another thing I wonder about is what would my life be like if I had married somebody who bought us a renovated farmhouse here on the Chesapeake Bay?

Thursday, August 5, 1971

I've just come back from playschool where I picked up the boys. I dropped Freddy and Gregory off and brought Thomas home. It's a beautiful day. This morning, I was out with the children, and Katherine threw a ball out in the street. When I went out in the street to get it, I fell and slightly hurt my knee. I don't think that I hurt myself as far as the baby is concerned, but I feel a little peculiar.

Sunday, we're going to a champagne party for Claire, and Frank told me to get a semblance of a tan so that I'd look tanned on Sunday. I will try to go out into the sun shortly.

Katherine went to sleep about one in the afternoon, and Frank went to work and took the children to playschool first. I called Zoe because she had called me to ask about the Outer Banks of North Carolina. We talked for about an hour, and by the time I finished, it was almost time to get Thomas. I wanted to record.

It's so strange: the difference between a day like today—when Frank left at one and took Thomas with him, Katherine went right to sleep, and I have a bit of space—and a day like last Tuesday, for example—Katherine took no nap at all. Frank didn't go to work until about two. If Katherine wakes up before I get Thomas in the house and if Frank goes to work late, I don't have any time for myself, and I desperately need it.

I saw in a book on parenthood or motherhood, which I just happened to pick up, that a mother should save something for herself, a little bit of herself for herself, and I think that's true. And the time that I have each day to myself is the little bit of time that I have saved for myself.

Shortly after my birthday, Frank took me downtown, and we had lunch at Freddy Martin's, and then we came back here. Frank's parents watched the children. The birthday lunch was very pleasant, and when we got back, his parents had gifts for us. Frank's parents gave me a beautiful handbag, and they gave Frank a tool kit. All in all, it was an enjoyable day although it had been a very busy one because I'd been to Dr. Kuhn's in the morning and Frank had been to the Y to take Thomas for his swimming lesson. After Frank's parents left, Mrs. Fisk came over, and I wanted to give her a check. I had told Frank so many times that she was coming. I went out to him and asked him for the check. He grumbled and asked Mrs. Fisk for a receipt. It's strange, his reactions. I don't remember now exactly what else he said, but it's things like that I don't understand. I had told him, and I thought we had agreed on all this, but he went on about it and said, "You'd better tell her not to do any more typing," as if I were extracting something from him. I said, "Frank, we had agreed on this and had it all worked out that once a week, I was going to give her a check." In the end, he went to the bank and took $150 out of savings account and put it into the checking account. I guess he figured that some of that money was mine. I felt hurt about the way he did that. When I thought about it though, I said to myself, "Well, forget it, because it's just one of the strange ways that he reacts. Frank went into a funk as if he were really being pushed for this check. He made me ask, and he gave it to me grudgingly as if I had sprung it on him at the spur of the moment, which I had made every effort not to do. I was upset about that at the end of an otherwise nice day.

Jane Smith came to see us with two of her girlfriends, Lorie and Roseanne. It always seems to me strange when I haven't seen somebody for a very long time, and then when I see that person, along with a couple of other people whom I don't know, I always feel that's a slight barrier because I can't talk exclusively to the one person. She stayed for a couple of hours and left. They were going to go out to the airport and pick up Jane's dog. She had some jewelry that she had been making, which she showed us. It was silver and blue wire hoop jewelry. She plans to go to Florida Presbyterian in the fall. It was strange, but I was sad when she left. The three girls went down over the lawn and got in the car and left, and I suddenly had an immensely sad feeling. It was inexplicable. It grabbed me. I didn't really expect it. It wasn't a very emotional time. It wasn't a spectacular visit in any way. But suddenly, in a flash, what came back to me was the time that she was here before, last summer, for about five days and the time that she was supposed to be picked up here by Pam and then dropped off at Frank's office where she was going to be picked up by Cecil. As it turned out, she never got picked up by Pam, so when I put Thomas in for his nap, I drove her to Frank's office. I took Katherine in the car and drove Jane to Frank's office.

As soon as she left, I came back and felt very sad. I couldn't figure out why. I don't know whether it was because I never really expressed to Jane some of the things that I wanted to tell her, or perhaps, she represents something to me, perhaps a young creative side or a kind of wholeness. She is probably one of the few people that I could have imagined being in my present life and being very happy. She's so complete in herself that she doesn't need restaurants or Georgetown to enhance her. I don't know what it was. Her father died only four years ago, and she said that her childhood all ended in one day. Maybe, it made me think about my own father's death. I don't understand what the association was, but the feelings that I had last summer came back in a flash. That night, Frank found it almost a strain when she called on the phone and said that they were coming, and when the three of them came, Thomas was awake, and he got fantastically rambunctious. He was wild, jumping all around the place. Katherine was asleep, and I kept thinking I should wake her up because she'll be awake all night otherwise. The sun began to flood the living room, and one of Jane's girlfriends kept making phone calls. That night, Frank told me he thought I was cross with the children and that he wondered whether I was happy in my role; I felt hurt about that. I went downtown to Carol Ann's and got my haircut, and Mandy watched the children. It was very strange; when I do anything like that, I always, toward the end, begin to get more and more frantic to come home and make sure the children are okay. But Carol Ann told me that she was going to take a job at night tending bar to help pay her bills. I had a feeling that she was a little depressed. I don't know how they are doing financially, but she gave me a nice haircut. Mandy said that she's decided to put her baby up for adoption.

Saturday night, Frank was angry or distant. It was very late before the children went to bed, and they woke up during the night. Sunday, Frank's parents came for dinner. I felt worked to death, but we've had many pleasant moments this week.

Yesterday, we went downtown, and I bought a bonny a-frame for the woodcut that Jane made for Thomas, and we bought some black cups in the Store, and I bought a dress. Frank helped me pick it out. I also bought a very open-weave knitted blouse. We stopped in a shop that carries wood hatch. They had a rosewood burl on the wall that was beautiful. It reminded me of Nakashima, and it reminded me of my father. Both were woodworkers. It was fascinating to see it.

I was telling Frank last night how much I wanted to do something creative, how much I wanted to write, and when I see something like

Nakashima's or Kepes's work, I want to do something like that. Then I begin to think that I can live my life without respect to money.

Last night, we came home, and I tried on my new things. Frank found some puppets in the Store, and we showed Thomas the puppets. We got quite a few things and had a nice time. It was immensely stimulating just to be down in Georgetown and walk around. We got back, and the children had had long naps, so they didn't miss us too much. I talked a lot to Frank, and I felt close to him and happy.

I looked back on the way I had felt Sunday. I felt resentful. Frank was sitting down reading Mario Puzo's *The Godfather*, and I had to go from one thing to the next. Then the children . . . I didn't have five minutes to myself. He has so much free time, and he's the first one to be tired, and he's the first one to think that he's got to go to the office. He thinks that because I don't have to go to an office, I have an easy life with nothing to do. Even though this feeling was welling up in me, I told myself not to feel that way because when I feel resentful, it's not only that I feel that way, but I also feel so unloving. I really want to love. I do want to feel that feeling, and last night, I felt so close to Frank and so happy, and the house looked so nice, and the frame looked so great. I felt fantastically happy. I liked the dress that I got, and Frank was so nice to me. He listened to the things I had to say. I was telling him that when I saw that big piece of rosewood on the wall, I thought it was so beautiful and that I want to create things.

I've been thinking about the difference between being in a personal atmosphere and in an impersonal atmosphere. To me, it's fascinating. I think that after a while, after you have children and you're home and in the house all day long, you begin to feel more detached, and this helps me feel freer.

Thursday, August 12, 1971

Frank left for work at 1:00 p.m., and I took Thomas, Freddy, and Gregory to playschool. I'm going to go down and pick them up at 3:00 p.m. Katherine Louise is sleeping. This is the first time that I have had a chance to do any recording for a few days, and it's great. It seems as though the past few times that I've tried to do something, either Katherine has not taken her nap or something has come up. It's really very hard to do anything even when Joan is here. I guess because the kids are in and out, in and out, and in and out.

I have to be by myself to record. It is a very pleasant spot in my day, especially when there have been several days when I haven't been able to record.

This morning, we went over to a fruit stand and bought all kinds of wonderful things—lettuce, tomatoes, cucumbers, onions, plums, peaches, grapes, and melons. The ride there was beautiful. It had rained last night and cleared the skies. The ride home this morning was gorgeous. We went all through the Agricultural Research Center and down by the Patuxent Wildlife Refuge area and then home.

This morning, when I was up and making the children's breakfast, the house looked beautiful. The autumn light is exquisite in the morning, and the air is cooler now. I can keep the windows and the doors open; it's delightful. When it's dead hot, the heat is so heavy it's like a weight that sits on your shoulders. But today, there is very low humidity, and the rain has made everything shiny, and the air is clear and the visibility good.

Last night, I washed the green bottle that I have on the windowsill over the sink, and as I was eating my lunch with Frank and the children, the bottle gleamed. Colored glass is fascinating, especially when you can see through it to see where there are leaves that move; it's intriguing.

Last night, I cleaned up the kitchen extra well. The bottle was one of the things that got washed, and I like the house so much more when it's really clean. I feel happy; I feel so incredibly happy. I don't understand how my moods can change so much. Today, I feel so happy when I look at the green glass bottle and look out the window at the leaves moving and with sunshine on them. Sitting in the living room and looking out at the view across the street, it looks so beautiful, and there is just enough wind so the leaves are moving, making a moving screen. I think it must have something to do with the pregnancy and being past the first three months, which is a very blah time. I felt so tired. Now, I feel fantastically happy, and I'm very happy to have this baby. I don't think that I want any more children beyond this though. I'm sure that I don't. Two seems almost too perfect. I began to wonder whether it could be that when you're pregnant, everything you look at also seems pregnant; everything seems resplendent with life. Everything looks cozy or warm or living. Everything has a spark of creation to it. From my experience, after Thomas was born, and also after Katherine, I was more aware of it after Thomas because I found it so shocking. I anticipated it more after Katherine was born. The images that went through my mind were images of destruction. When I looked out the window, what I saw was decay. When I glanced up at the ceiling or the wall, what I saw were the cracks, signs of disintegration and decay everywhere. Whereas during pregnancy, everything that I see seems full of life. It's creation overflowing.

It's such a great joy to have time to myself. Everyone needs some time to oneself, but to be as busy as I am and then to have little spots of time is very nice, especially when one is not tired or harried for any reason. Right now, having time to myself on a beautiful day makes me feel extra happy. But I also feel fantastically free. I don't feel that this baby is going to tie me down. I feel incredibly free, and I have increasingly felt that way; maybe, it's true that each child you have is another chance at perfection.

I feel that I'm in high school, as though the next thing I'm going to do is start planning my career. That's how I feel. It's crazy. I suppose that's how people who've been previously married feel when they remarry at age seventy. It's a feeling that anything is possible. It's hard for me to imagine being depressed for long. My biggest complaint is being tired and harried and impatient. Basically, I feel free and happy; I feel I can do anything I want to do, which is strange. I feel that life is wonderful. It's full of joy and happiness. I feel now like running out the front door and dancing down the street. I feel like singing a hymn to creation.

After Thomas was born, I realized I was not free; eventually, this changed, and now, I feel so much freer than I felt before I was married or after, for that matter, freer than probably any time in my life. Maybe, there are certain things in my nature that are being fulfilled. There isn't any sort of longing, any deep, subterranean longing. I feel fulfilled, and I can do anything. I am immensely free and immensely happy. I feel a profound natural happiness.

I was thinking how peculiar it is that things can change so much; I can look at the very same view—that is, the view from my living room window—and think there are times when I've thought it's even boring to look at. There was a time at the beginning of this pregnancy when I felt that way. Then there are other times when I can look out at it and think, "Isn't that the most beautiful view I have ever seen in my whole life?" It's strange that things can change so much, such as moods and feelings about people and places.

I'm really glad that I have become increasingly fond of this house. I guess my moods now alternate between that and occasionally feeling very annoyed with Frank. I don't know why.

One day after swimming, we drove up Colstone Road, and we went past Dr. Sil's office, which was impressive from the outside. That was the day Frank took me downtown for lunch on my birthday. When we came back late that evening, Hettie Fisk came over with the typing, and I was so annoyed with Frank because at that moment, he called up Jane Smith, and I had to ask him for the check, and he acted so grumpy. It made me furious because I had been over this with him before and we had agreed that I would get the typing done and, naturally, pay the woman for doing the typing. So many times, he pulls a funk, either if I invite somebody over without consulting him first or if I venture out on my own. It reminds me of the time before Thomas was born when people would call me up long-distance from Boston, not very often, but once in a while. Frank would just go on and on and on. He felt so intruded upon when that call came right then. It was always at what he thought was the most inconvenient time. And it always seemed to me so strange because it wasn't a strange time; it wasn't 2:00 a.m. I'd feel bad, guilty, as though I wanted to make it up to him. It still surprises me when things like this happen, and they usually happen when we have company. I don't know why. There's a pattern to it. I was angry to think that he was so ungracious about it. I've got to realize what it is that I want and then, if I do want to have something, realize that if he acts that way, well, he is perfectly entitled to act that way. All I can do is not to get that involved or angry, but just try to be reasonable and fair and say, "Well, if you want somebody to come some other time, or if you want me to arrange it differently, I can arrange it differently."

My sister, Louise, is coming here tomorrow, and Frank saw the time of her arrival. He thought it was an inconvenient time as if he has a very rigid schedule. He acts so imposed upon, especially if there's anything before noon. It's almost beyond him. That annoyed me. Looking back at it now, it had grown a little vague in my mind, but I felt angry, absolutely furious. We had come back from downtown, his parents had taken care of the children, and we came home, and I made a meal. We all sat down and ate, and the kids seemed especially unruly and fussy. Frank's parents had lovely gifts for us, a handbag for me and a toolbox for Frank. Then after they left, Mrs. Fisk came, and then after she left, I had the two children get ready for bed. Meanwhile, all this time, Frank didn't have anything to do. There are a lot of things he could do; he seems to have so much more time than I do. Watching the children—imagine the number of hours I have to spend every day just watching them—along with all the other things to be done, is tiring, and for him to act in that manner was awful. But we did have a very nice time before that. We bought a big white pot, which sits on the floor, and it'll be fun to put a big plant or ficus tree in it.

Jane Smith came with two friends and visited us one day. The only thing about it that was interesting was that when Jane left, I had exactly the same emotional reaction as when she left after she had stayed with us last summer. In the strangest way, I had total recall of that whole experience last summer. And thinking it over, I was amazed that we did as much as we did. We saw the movie *Z*, and we went down to the playground and to the stables in Kettering and to the National Gallery, and Frank and I went to see the *Tropic of Cancer*. She babysat for us the other night. It was amazing. Also, at that time, I didn't have time to breathe, really didn't have time to breathe. Katherine was about nine or ten months old. But to have this exact same emotional response, I felt very sad, the same sadness I felt before. I don't understand why. Looking at it from a Jungian point of view, I would say that she must represent an avenue to something that I want to find in myself, and when she left, it was as if that avenue left too. I guess she represents something creative to me. It was unusual to have that exact same response again.

Mandy Parkland babysat for us, and I guess she's going to have her baby in the first part of September. She says she will have it adopted.

Last Wednesday, Frank and I went downtown and bought a bonny a-frame for Jane's print. I absolutely love it. I could carry it around from room to room with me. I keep it out in the kitchen although it's really intended for Thomas's room. We had a tremendously good time when we went downtown. I bought a dress that Frank helped me pick out, which I wore to the champagne party on Sunday for Claire Smith and Jim Roberts. We went into the Hot Shoppes for hamburgers, and outside, there was a brand-new Cadillac. There was a little sign, a little bigger than the license plate, that said, "The Episcopal Church welcomes you." After a while, there were three or four hippy-looking kids sitting on it. It was so funny.

The stores down in Georgetown looked great, and I got anxious to buy some things for fall and to buy some things for the baby after it is born. I saw some great clothes at Joe's Place and at the Airport. I love winter and autumn clothes. That made me feel great. We also went into the Baycraft place that sells wooden pieces, some of them are tables made from hatch doors. But there are other things too, things made from driftwood and some regular things made from wood. I saw the most fantastic rosewood burl on a white wall. It was exquisite, and I think I've already covered this a little bit, but I thought of the furniture maker Nakashima and the artist Kepes. It's something that Jane Smith would really appreciate. People who can make things like that are fantastic. That's what I want to do in writing if I possibly can.

That night, when we came home, Frank and I had a long talk, one of these fabulous talks where our conversation is like stepping stones, about my childhood home and how it would have looked if it had white walls and simpler, more classic, almost-Amish type of furniture and if my father had made more of the furniture there and then the rest of the furnishings had come from Design Research. It is strange to think of my parents' life in light of that. I think that's such a key thing about my mother's personality, and as Frank said, "Look where she lives now." You can see the way she relates to her environment. I'm still responding to what those vibrations meant or didn't mean. It's the very opposite of something like May Sarton's *Plant Dreaming Deep.*

My mother sent me an absolutely beautiful greeting card from the Fine Arts Museum in Boston. It's a reproduction of a painting of Mt. Vernon Street in Boston by Alfred Clifton Goodwin. I had never seen it before, and I love it. My sister sent me a postcard of Louisburg Square, saying what time she's going to arrive. I don't know why, but there's something about looking at pictures or looking at things that I find infinitely satisfying. It's as though a whole dream landscape opens up. I want to see some external representation of my internal world. I guess that I've never expressed myself, and I find such an urge to do this. I feel that I can do that here, as well as anyplace else. I do think that now.

I don't know if I could feel any happier if I were in a deckhouse or if I lived on Capitol Hill or Georgetown or Louisburg Square.

On Sunday, we went to Claire's party. It was at Ruth and Frank Tooker's house in Virginia. I had a good time. I had to imagine what a good time I have on some of these little excursions. The difference between my life now and my life before marriage, when I lived in Boston, is that now, my life has much more of a center. Before, my life had more of a periphery. It was interesting to meet Claire's new husband. I think he's financially very successful. If there was anything Claire found lacking in her marriage to Bud Smith, it was that they didn't have money, and it's almost as though she's got a chance to be her own daughter. She has a chance to find what she wants in a second marriage, which was missing in her first marriage. I think she's found it, and I think that it is strange because she's found it at a time when she probably has enough money between her father's death, her husband's death, and her mother-in-law's death. All these people left her quite a bit of money. It's really strange she is marrying somebody with money just at the point when she doesn't have to do that. It saves her daughters, Pam and Jane, from having to go through financially advantageous marriages.

The house was charming in a way, but it was not air-conditioned and had too much furniture. It may have been the heat and the fact that there were a lot of people there, but if it had about half the number of furniture that it had in it, it would be exquisite, absolutely exquisite. There was greenery all around it. You thought you were out in the woods. Everywhere you looked, there were green leaves. Art Stover came over, but Frank said afterward he was probably high. I didn't hear all of it because I had to get out for some reason. But Art Stover was telling Frank how he really liked the Chesapeake Bay for boating and how he really liked to go boating. And what he would like to do is to buy a cottage and use it for vacations and weekends and then retire there. But his wife didn't like it because she didn't like fisherman types. She didn't think they were very classy. The Stovers moved to Potomac because they thought it was a more socially upscale community than Cheverly, and we went to their house about a year ago. They had a party in the basement and kept everybody in the basement. It reminded me of high school when you have a party in the basement and you don't want your parents to butt in on it. Anyway, after I had heard these people had moved to Potomac, which is the second-nicest place in this whole area to live in, we went out there, and I thought, "What a completely sterile place." My reaction to that was the same as my reaction to Hettie and Alfred's house. How sterile, how utterly sterile. It's like an instant house. There are several sets of furniture. Each room has a set of furniture and accessories. Fran Stover seems like a very hard person, but it's probably because she's from Texas or her manner of speaking or her outward veneer. Art Stover gives you a picture that what he really likes to do is mess around with boats and wear old clothes while his wife is dying to go out; and if they do not go out, she's trying to always push, push, push for more financial success. Frank mentioned afterward, "I think Art Stover is a salt-of-the-earth type of guy, a warmhearted guy, and certainly mor warmhearted than she is." It was like a stereotypical suburban story: the wife trying to push her husband all the time and all he wants to do is play in the basement while she's going out of her mind trying to get all these unfulfilled things fulfilled. It's such an incredible stereotype. If anything points to the theory that marriage is on the way out, it's that. The party was interesting. These people don't know that's what's wrong with marriage. I have a feeling that probably, Bud and Claire's marriage was something like that, except that Claire is much more on the ball than Fran Stover, also she smiles and laughs a lot more, has more fun, and enjoys herself more. She's got high spirits and is young, so that's why you're not aware of this other side. I guess that she is finding in her new marriage all the financial things that she didn't have in her old marriage. What's really strange is that Claire has put a tremendous effort into finding a new husband who would be suitable. She's had plastic surgery on her face, and maybe, I'm just a stick in the mud; maybe, it's sour grapes. To me, her face has no expression; from her mouth upward, there's no expression there at all. It's like a mask, and the tan is so heavy that it makes her skin look like leather. Also, it looks as though her skin is pulling away from her eyes. It's amazing that she put all her effort into recreating the same kind of existence. When I look at women like Anna or Connie Starr, I think these women are more self-directed. I see so many women like Claire, so anxious to get into this suburban life. It's hard to imagine that anybody would want it that badly. It's much easier for me to understand somebody like Connie Starr than it is for me to try to understand somebody like Claire. She always said that she wanted to play the organ, and it surprises me that she didn't take music lessons or do something like that on her own or for herself, or take a trip to Europe.

Frank's mother and father babysat for us, and when we came back from Claire's party, we stopped at the Hot Shoppe, just for the air-conditioning, and to have a cup of coffee. It was the Key Bridge Hot Shoppe, almost on the Virginia side of Georgetown. It was very attractive. They had a moat around the building, and every couple of yards, there was a fountain of water. It was extremely pleasant. Then when we did come home, Frank's mother had put both the children into bed. When I left, they were both napping, so it was from 1:00 p.m. until we went to bed, say around midnight, that I wasn't the one taking care of the children. When my mind is not occupied with the children, it can roam far afield. It's amazing. It's fantastic, and I began to feel that I should wake the children up since it had been so long since I'd seen them.

Frank and I had a fight Sunday night. We stopped at the Hot Shoppe, had mentioned that when my sister came down, maybe we could or breakfast, and then coming home, he suggested maybe we should spend the weekend at the Madison Hotel. When we got home, I told Frank I thought I'd call up Claire and ask her and Jim to come over some night. Frank said he didn't think that the house looked good enough, that he thought we should buy a plant for the pot that we bought at the Store, that maybe we should buy a new chrome lamp, and that maybe he should paint the living room. I said maybe we should get some drapes. That just changed the whole thing, the mention of the word "drapes." He said that I never took finances into account and asked me if I was aware that he had only so many dollars in his checking account and only so many dollars in the office account and if I was not aware of this and why I was always mentioning these extravagant things.

Monday night, I felt the baby move. I was amazed because this is the fourth month. Tuesday night, I felt the same thing. I found it so hard when Frank was saying that he's thinking about increasing his insurance for me, that all the money that's spent on clothes in this house is spent on me, that I eat very well, and that all the money is spent on me, and that I never pay any attention to finances. I said, "Well, it's very hard for me to have a picture of what the finances are because I don't have any kind of financial frame to work in." It was horrible. The minute I mentioned drapes, Frank said I wasn't aware of his finances, and he went through his whole financial picture. I just clammed up, and he said to me, "What? Did I say something wrong? I mean you look so hurt." It was then that I said, "Well, the reason I clam up is because if I say anything that expresses any initiative at all, you clamp right down on me, and I may as well not talk. I might as well just say yes or no to whatever you say." I said I don't want a relationship like that, where there are things that are taboo. That's when he started to say that all the money that's spent here is spent on me. I was annoyed. There is a pattern to this, and he had mentioned weekending at the Madison and all these other expensive things. Granted that he didn't mean them, still, it was all in the same vein. I was furious; I was absolutely furious. Frank doesn't carry on any kind of an argument. When something like that comes up, he doesn't see that as an opportunity to clear the air or for greater understanding. He thinks it is a tragedy that at the end of a day, this should happen. Very soon afterward, he picked up the newspaper and read it. I was left with a strange feeling. The Dick Cavett Show was on, and it was so stupid to waste my time listening to it. I had finished reading *Up the Sandbox* and hadn't started anything else, and I was thinking, "I wish I were into a book so I could pick it up and read." But it always happens when I'm irritated. I want to go on and on and on about it. It's hard for me then to switch off and start reading a newspaper. Frank does that very easily. In fact, that is his defense. He always does that. I'm sitting there ready to fight, but I'm left with this furious up-in-the-air feeling, and I feel too angry and too full of fight to go to sleep. There isn't anything that I can get into as far as reading, and I'm angry at myself for wasting this precious time I've had since noontime without the children, and here I am arguing with Frank. At the time, I feel so furious, and that's what's wrong with marriage. Yet today, I just couldn't feel happier.

I do feel tremendously happy when I was telling Frank about Mandy Parkland and her decision to keep the baby. I was telling Frank what Mandy told me about her father—how he had hurt her mother, how upset her mother was by his drinking, how her mother had tried to help him but had finally given up, and how Mandy, a couple of times, said she had hated her father, but she didn't hate him anymore, she just felt sorry for him. When I was telling Frank this, Frank said, "Well, you figure the guy had four kids and suddenly he realized, probably at the age of forty because Mandy said that he never drank much as a teenager or a young man in his twenties and it was only something like ten years ago he started to drink, and all of a sudden that was it. He was just an alcoholic." Frank said, "For him, the American dream all his life was that success was just around the corner. And then all of a sudden, he realized that it's not going to happen, and he was going to go on and on. Life isn't going to get any better; in fact, it's probably going to get worse. You're physically going to go downhill, and your ability to work is probably going to go downhill, and you are saddled with a wife and family and a house and cars, and all you can look forward to is the payments that you're going to be making, and you never will make a million dollars—you never will be a success." I think that is probably true. He was like that, and I thought of our friend Phil and how much Phil was like that. And probably, also my grandfather. He started drinking, and I wonder if it's not that men who are like this all brutalize their inner nature and that when their dream of success or other dreams begin to collapse and their fantasy gets farther and farther away from reality, they either crack up or become alcoholics. However, those who are married have payments to make. The difference between the ones that plod along and the ones that don't, I suppose, is that the ones that manage not to go off the deep end are the ones that do have some kind of an inner life to sustain them. When you see Phil, you realize that he's just a shell. But it's interesting to think of that in light of Art Stover. He sounded as though he's about ready to hit the open road, except for this woman who is after him to buy more insurance and symbols of affluence and success.

I think it's really true that you have to have your own revolution. I sense that a lot of people think I should push Frank, but in myself, I do feel that all his life, he's been so used to being pushed that in order for him to do anything, he still needs to be pushed, but I really don't want to do that. It was strange about that argument. I decided that in order to argue and fight, you need time. The same road can lead to something creative or else something destructive. I felt horrible because on Sunday night, imagine having this little bit of free time and then spending it in such a stupid way. Maybe, I did make some point to Frank. I know you have to spend some time talking things over, but it seems so painful. Another Sunday, when his parents came over, when we had a birthday cake to celebrate Frank's birthday, I recall that from the moment I got up, I just worked, worked, worked. While I was getting the dinner, taking care of the children, making a cake, and getting ready to go out, he just sat down and read the whole time. And then when he tells me he wonders whether I am happy in my role because I seem a little cross with the children, which is what he told me one night, it makes me absolutely furious. I feel that what he's saying makes no sense at all. Not only that, but I have to have my own standards because if I had his standards for me, I would just work, work, work all the time and then be criticized for being tired or cross with the children. I absolutely have to have my own standards, absolutely, and do my own thing. That's one thing that my experience with Frank has taught me. I can't give up one side of my nature for another side of either my own nature or for somebody else's nature. I think that's such a valuable lesson. Every now and then, I think of what my life would have been like if I hadn't given up my job at MIT but had married Frank or somebody else and had children in Boston.

When I think of women like that woman in Vermont, which I so often think about, or Beverly Bloomberg's mother, who spent all her time trying to, almost like propaganda, convince you that she is superior to her mate. "You know, he's only Mr. Bloomberg, but me, I'm a Backman." The woman in Vermont said about her husband, "He is such a stupid minister that the only church that he could be assigned to is this one in Rutland, Vermont, whereas I'm so cultured that I'm the only one in the whole of Rutland that has a copy of a book by Ferlinghetti." There's a difference between you just standing there and criticizing your mate because he doesn't fulfill your other side and you finding out what area is available to you and then claiming it, doing something about it, being as creative as you possibly can within the area that is open to you, within the little spot that you have for yourself. The difference is that women like Mrs. Bloomberg or like Mrs. Vermont have a little ego that spends all its time trying to defend itself. Whereas if it embraced more, it would be infinitely enlarged.

There was a woman at the champagne party on Sunday who was from Massachusetts. First, she said Plymouth and Taunton; then she said she grew up in Cambridge between Central Square and Harvard Square. She said she liked living here much better than in Massachusetts. I said, "Well, I guess you would like a small town better than living in a county." She said to me, "Have you ever lived in a small town?" and I said, "No." She said I'd probably be unhappy in a small town. I was thinking about the description of the small town, thinking of it in terms of its architecture and history. I was thinking of Northumberland, Pennsylvania, where Hettie and Alfred lived, about Frank's description of this town and the fact that Frank thinks the reason Mandy and Robb are the way they are is because of this small town. It's just like that book review today for *Craig and Joan* by Elliott Asimoff. It was as much a story of a town, the fact that this town wanted so much to repress the channels for allowing young people to express their better instincts, their more humanitarian instincts. After this couple kill themselves, the town proceeds to minimize the impact of the suicide. The town officials said, "Well, there must have been some other reason for their doing that." I guess that's an example of a small town. I think it was in New Jersey. I suppose you can get into a small town, like Peyton Place, that is really completely corrupt. I do want to feel that I am open to new experiences and that somehow, I can use my experiences creatively, but I guess that if you do marry or live closely with somebody, what you can have is a kind of enlargement that you otherwise might not have.

Katherine has just about learned to talk. And the past two days, it's been very exciting. She has now learned to say, "I want," and she says, "I want to wear this," and "I want to wear that." Thomas said to me yesterday, "Where's Daddy?" And Katherine said, "Where's Daddy?" And I looked at her, trying to have her repeat it, and I said "Where's Daddy?" And she said, "I don't know." And she says, "I want ice cream." It's really fantastic. She's really grown up in the past week; yesterday, it was raining, and in the late afternoon about four, I noticed that she was playing in the house. For the very first time, I was able to get a meal without constantly having her either underfoot, pulling everything out of the cupboard, climbing up trying to get into the sink, getting up on the kitchen table or the purple cabinet, or else, having Thomas start hitting her. She just played and played, and I thought, "Thank goodness she's almost two." I think that period from one to two is so difficult, especially when the child starts walking and you have to watch its every step and the child is into everything. In the past week, she's really grown up quite a bit. And she's utterly adorable. She wakes up in the morning and calls, "Daddy and Mommy, Daddy and Mommy." And Frank pointed out that Thomas used to say, "Mommy and Daddy, Mommy and Daddy," which is true.

Last night, we saw a TV program on the blues musician Lightning Hopkins, and it showed some scenes of where he came from, somewhere in the south. It was fantastic to see this utterly poor community, a little place, and the most unbelievable thing was when they showed the main street—it had parking meters on it. They had parking meters every three feet. Frank pointed it out, and I thought, "I never quite made that connection." Once he said it, I thought, "My God, what an unbelievable commentary on that place, to see the parking meters. It looked to me as though that place had no electricity, and I doubt if they had underground wires, and there were no telephone poles. It looked as though they had no telephones, no electricity. Frank mentioned that in one of these places, he saw a whole lot of black-eyed susans growing in the midst of this poverty.

Tuesday, August 17, 1971

Katherine is napping, Thomas is at playschool, and Frank is at the office. Last night, we took my sister and her five-year-old son, Gary, to the airport. They came down Friday morning and left last night.

I think that I have reached a good point in my pregnancy because I feel so incredibly happy. Everything makes me happy. I feel free. I feel that I can do anything that I want. I feel as though this is another chance at perfection.

I was struck by the realization that I don't see any images of decay, whereas previously, most of the time, if I looked, for instance, out the window, I saw papers strewn on the street, and I would think, "What will happen? There will be more and more of them," and whenever an appliance broke, it seemed like the end of the world, as though there is increasing decay, breakdown, or fragmentation. I guess it's because I feel so attached to my environment that when anything is broken, dirty, cracked, or battered, I feel it too. I don't see anything like that now. When I'm outside or in the car and I see the countryside around here, it looks beautiful, especially on Central Avenue and toward Upper Marlboro. It appears fantastically beautiful. Creation is everywhere, and I don't see destruction anywhere. I have more energy too, and it's wonderful not to feel completely exhausted. Katherine Louise is getting a little bit easier to take care of, at least in the house.

The past eight months or so, it had been difficult to take care of her because of that year-and-a-half stage when there's no way to discipline a child and I have to be with her constantly.

Mrs. Fisk said if she typed the whole motherhood work, she would charge $1.50 per page instead of $1.75. I asked my sister, when she was here, what kind of typewriter Mother has, and she said she still has that little portable that I got when I graduated from high school. We may go to Boston in September, and I may take the typing up there with me. Maybe, I'll leave some of it with Mother and see if she'd like to do it. Maybe, I'll ask her to type it.

Mrs. Adams finally came. She had skipped on Monday, but she finally called me and came another Monday. It was a week ago yesterday, and she worked from morning until about 5:00 p.m. I hope that she continues to come. Joan's been coming a little bit, which is a help. Those two things do make it a little bit easier, and Katherine is at a slightly easier age. Each time I have a guest here, I realize that even though there are times when I feel terribly crowded and squeezed in, I think of how I have felt at other times, and I realize that it's much easier now than it was before. I don't think it could ever be that hard again.

I talked to my friend Zoe on the phone a couple of times. She and Myron are thinking of going to Nag's Head, and she was asking me about it. She is a homebody par excellence.

In some ways, it gets a little easier to have people here because I can just enjoy being here with them. I don't feel as though I have to go someplace or take them someplace quite as much, especially if it's somebody that I enjoy talking to. It's quite nice to have people here.

My sister, Louise, came on Friday and brought her son, Gary, with her, and Thomas and Gary got along well, considering Gary is two years older. They played very well. Gary was aggressive toward Frank at times, but I think it has something to do with his father. Frank found it a little disturbing. Gary talked constantly about his father. It's very sad. Louise said that her ex-husband doesn't seem to have any idea what a big thing divorce is for Gary. One of the last times that his father came to see them, Gary cried and cried and begged his father to stay. His father was annoyed and accused my sister of putting Gary up to it, putting him up to this dramatic plea for his father to stay at home with them.

On Friday, we came back here and relaxed and sat outside in the afternoon after lunch, and Joan came and watched Katherine a little bit. In the evening, Paul Lister came over for dinner, and we had a nice dinner of corn on the cob and ham. But I couldn't get Katherine to sleep. One time, when she was up, she got a peanut from the table, and I didn't realize when I put her into bed that it was still in her mouth. She started to choke on it, and as a result, she threw up. It was a nightmare, not being able to get this little one to bed, but still, it didn't seem as bad as some previous occasions like that.

We had wine with dinner and talked. Paul talked mostly about computers and the work that he was doing, and he seemed to be quite proud of his work and liked it very much. I was a little bit worried about Katherine Louise because it seemed that she just coughed and coughed, and then Thomas started coughing too.

Saturday, Frank went to work, and originally, Frank said that maybe we ought to ask his parents to come over or get a babysitter and take my sister out on Saturday night. But it seemed to me it would be more fun to go to Georgetown during the day on Saturday and go to some of the stores because I remember when we went there before, my sister seemed interested in looking in the stores. Frank came home at 2:00 p.m., and we left for Georgetown. My sister had given up drinking coffee, and most of the time, she eats quickly and is all finished and ready to go. I can't quite keep up with her. I'm always busy either with dishes or fixing a meal or taking care of a baby. But Saturday, we went to Georgetown, and Frank minded the children. My sister took a nap before we went there. I enjoyed myself immensely, just walking around and looking at things. My sister didn't seem quite as keen on looking in the stores. But we bought her daughter, Lois, some flowers, and I found a little Arabia pitcher at the Store. We went to an ice cream parlor and sat out in the garden and had some ice cream. I just felt great. For the first time, I could really relax with my sister. Before, she seemed nervous. It wasn't so much that she wanted to do anything or go anyplace in particular, but she seemed nervous, whereas this time, I wondered if things were too dull; maybe, we should have gotten up and rushed out someplace. She seemed perfectly content to sit on the sofa. I don't know why. She told me that our house was comfortable, and she seemed quite content not to go anywhere. I did ask her if there was any place special that she wanted to go. We spent hours and hours and hours talking. We had plenty of time.

There have been times when my friend Connie had come to visit, and during which, either I have made more elaborate meals or we've done many different things so that I absolutely never had a chance to talk to her.

We came back here at about 7:00 p.m., and Katherine Louise was already in bed, and she slept all through the night. This made my life much easier. We had stopped at the Emporium and got paper kites for Thomas and Gary. I took my sister into the Bay Craft Store and showed her a rosewood burl on the wall. On Sunday, we had dinner in the middle of the day, and then we went to Annapolis and took the three children with us. It was rather hot there, but we sat on benches for a while and watched the boats in the water. We went down on Central Avenue, Route 214, and the ride was beautiful, really exquisite. We drove back from Annapolis, picked up a copy of the *New York Times*, and took the kids to McDonald's, which the kids enjoyed to no end. It was a big relief for me. We came back here, and the boys watched *Sesame Street* and went to bed.

Frank was really ailing the whole weekend. He couldn't figure out whether he had a cold or his allergy. He felt ill and left work early on Saturday. I guess it's amazing that he was able to watch the children. But Sunday, we took the three kids out, so he had the place to himself for the afternoon. Just going to McDonald's and not having to cook dinner is a break. I found one McDonald's where we can sit and look out at the trees, so I don't find that unpleasant at all. The children were remarkably good, so it was possible for my sister and me to talk and watch the children too.

On Monday, I took them out to show them Holy Family Church. About 11:00 a.m., we went out in the car and ate at the Junior Hot Shoppes, which the kids absolutely adored. They had two milk shakes each. Then we drove to Upper Marlboro. The ride through these country roads just about blew my mind away.

After that, we rode to Upper Marlboro and back, and then we went to Watkins Park—the children loved the playground. Then we went into the snack bar and had some ice cream and then came home. Katherine Louise napped, and I cooked steak and made a salad, and we had ice cream. She just woke up at the right time to eat, and then we drove my sister and Gary to the airport. Frank came to the airport with us. He drove us there and back. When we came back from Watkins Park, before I got dinner, my sister and I sat out in the yard while Katherine was sleeping and the two boys were watching *Sesame Street*. It was very pleasant. We talked, my sister and I, just talked and talked and talked the whole time. I think she's doing very well. It's amazing when I think of her situation as compared to Claire's. It's amazing. I think that there is one respect in which she and I are both lucky, and that is Dorchester might have been a good place to live in. There is access to facilities there, much better than what some people have out in the suburbs. She's been accepted for the Licensed Practical Nurse (LPN) course at the Shattuck Hospital. It's for one year, but I think she's getting cold feet, and I tried to talk to her and tell her that she should take the course. I don't know whether she will. She should plan the whole year, sending the kids away on their school vacations and paying her neighbor Pat to come in the morning and getting as much off her back as she possibly can. She said she'd need a car. I think she's beginning to see how hard it will be to have to be there at seven in the morning in the winter. She quoted our sister-in-law Ruth as saying something like "Well, an LPN is not as good as an Registered Nurse (RN)." Another program, she's been thinking about, the Audwyn program does lead to an RN and takes three years. If she thinks it would be hard doing this at Shattuck for a year, it would be much harder for three years. It's true that an RN is better than an LPN, but Medical Doctor (MD) is better than RN. You could just go on and on. My sister and her husband are getting a divorce in October, and he's apparently going to contest the amount of money she wants. Other than that, they are both agreeing to get a divorce. It will be final in six months. What is so amazing to me is that she said that she always wanted to stay at home because going out and having a job or competing or going to college always seemed too difficult. She has the ideas in her head that our mother has told her, terrible things that have happened to people, like losing their jobs. My mother often said, "Oh, we'll probably go to the poor house," and our mother always used to say things to her like "If anything happens to your father, I don't know what I'd do." She had a feeling of incredible insecurity as a child, mostly financial insecurity. The prospect of going out and getting a job or adjusting to outer reality seemed overwhelming to her. Marriage was a way out. Her analyst said that she wanted to remain a child. She didn't go on to whatever that next step is in early adulthood, where you go from adolescence to adaptation to outer reality. She stayed at this one point, one level. This is unbelievably amazing for her to say because there is an inner world and an outer world. All my energies were directed to adapting to the outer world. It's what I guess was missing in Mother's life, and Mother is the same way. She's so beautifully adapted to the outer world, to being a career girl. Then marriage and motherhood threw her for such a loop that she never really saw any possibilities in it and was anxious to get out of it. The impression she gave me was that it was completely and totally wonderful to work and go out into the world as though the smartest thing a woman could do was jump in a car and drive off, not having to look left or right, not having to turn around at all, not even to wave goodbye, just zooming off straight ahead. But apparently, the impression my sister got was "If anything ever happened to your father . . ." People went out and got jobs, but they lost them, and terrible things always happened in the outside world. So my sister was encouraged to stay at this particular level. My mother's life was seesawing between these two things. I was forced out, and my sister was forced in. I think my mother did a beautiful job with "out" but a poor job with "in," and the things that my sister talked about I found interesting and pertinent to me as well. I guess that's probably why we talked so much. My sister talked and talked and talked. It was as though she was more interested in what she was saying than in what I was saying. Maybe, she wasn't, but she was more interested in talking and being heard. I found the whole thing quite interesting, but what's more interesting was this "in" and "out" idea.

There was an article in the *New York Times* that said that psychiatrists are now studying the phases of adult development, and there are as many stages of adult development that are as difficult to go through as it is from childhood to adolescence and adolescence to adulthood. This period of early adulthood is a period of adjustment to the outside world, to master the skills that one has to have in order to live. The other adjustment, at some point around thirty or maybe even older, is to begin to look for inner satisfaction. I think this is probably true. I think this is true with artists, who get their training and then begin to express what's really inside them. That's when some artists really appear to be original. Certainly, that's true with me. The way I felt about my education was that I never expressed anything of myself. My urge to express myself as I have gotten older has gotten stronger and stronger. I think the whole move from the city to Cherry Hill and then here have been related to that. For me, it's being weaned from the outside world so that I can concentrate on my own inner development. I think that with my sister, the reverse is true. At the end of our lives, we'll be evened out or equal.

It's interesting the things that she told me about some of the people around our old neighborhood—for example, that Smith is a bookie and that Freddy Flynn was in all kinds of trouble with, as she called them, the bone breakers, the loan sharks, because he was constantly gambling. Matt Glavin works for an insurance company, and his wife is a nurse in the delivery room at St. Margaret's Hospital. Talking about Sonny O'Higgins, Freddy Flynn, Smith, and all the people that she mentioned from around that area, I realized no one that she mentioned has ever done anything admirable. I don't know of anybody she mentioned that became a professional man. They are all semicrooked, running parking lots, and cheating on the take. Freddy Flynn has the same job his father had cutting the grass at the church. She talked about our old neighbors across the street and how her friend Lisa is very unhappy. She's been married a couple of years, she's a nurse, and she doesn't like her husband. She has one little boy, and she has a whole slew of family members who could take care of the child for her. She's got her sister, her cousin Denise, her other cousin Cathy, and her mother to take care of him. It sounds like an unbelievable desire to have a feast of masochism. It is as though Lisa were brought up where somebody was always mean to her, so she's recreated this same situation. All the people that my sister talks about, if they're apparently successful, it is in some petty crime.

Probably, in some ways, my sister was unable to appreciate my mother's good points. She was totally consumed by her own problems. She'd just as soon talk on in a gossipy way about everybody that she knows and about their lives. It's very interesting because we know so many people in common, because we are sisters, and we talk about our parents and our family. I think she's done a good job of integrating everything. She's quite strong in her own viewpoint, what she thinks about different people and what she thinks about that neighborhood. It is amazing. She has never been outside that neighborhood where we grew up. I think she's got a very good grip on her life, her life with her then-husband and the experience that she has just been through. I think she's lucky that she's going to her particular analyst. I hope I didn't give her too much advice. She tells a lot of funny stories about those people in our old neighborhood. She mentioned again that her husband had helped Dad paint the whole house just before Dad died and that her husband used to take Dad shopping and pick up Mother after work at the state hospital. We talked about the time when her husband was wallpapering the bathroom and Frank and I had driven up from Maryland to Boston. When we got there, we were amazed that he had gone to school all day, worked from three to eleven at the state hospital, then, at eleven, came home and was wallpapering the bathroom. He was having a hard time matching the paper. "You know," she said, "how fond my husband was of Dad," and I think that is true to some extent, but she mentioned again that Mother had said her husband killed Dad. That's just unbelievable. All those emotions in that house! All those people's mothers! My sister feels that our brother, David, turned my mother against my sister's ex-husband. It's strange that my mother should say that her ex-husband killed Dad when my sister thinks that her ex-husband helped Dad more than any one of our three brothers or more than our three brothers combined. All these things are disturbing to discuss.

The only thing that was slightly unpleasant about the whole time was that Frank didn't feel very well, and for whatever reasons, a cold or his hay fever, or maybe this was just an out for him, he did go over on Friday with us and get my sister, and then Paul Lister came, and that was nice because Frank suggested that we ask him. That seemed to work out well, and we had a nice dinner. He did mind the kids for us on Saturday, but it seemed that every time my sister and I were here, Frank was either in bed or else watching TV. He hardly talked to my sister. Maybe, I should blame myself because maybe, I didn't think of enough things to bring them together. But neither one of them made any effort to talk to the other. I think, maybe, Frank thinks my sister is hard to talk to. I don't know. But Sunday morning, it seemed there were a few things Frank could have done if he wanted to. He could have taken Thomas and Gary for a walk. There were moments that seemed difficult, such as getting dinner on Sunday and Katherine crying and Thomas wanting to take out his kite in the worst way, and I kept telling him, "But there is not enough wind." Finally, he took it out, and he accidentally ripped the tail off.

September 28, 1971

Every now and then, I have pangs of guilt about having left my motherhood manuscript with Connie and Anna. I wouldn't be surprised if Connie is furious in her manner because it is an imposition, and I'm sure that Connie will think that it sounds like her sister constantly complaining about what it's like to be a mother. I called the director of studies of the Jung Foundation. I have guts galore. Maybe, I have more purpose and less substance, but I do feel guilty about getting this motherhood diary typed. Curiously enough, I feel as though it's a waste of money. I guess I shouldn't feel that way. That's very strange. All these things make me feel slightly guilty. I also feel Frank might not approve because he might have to pay for it. But my goals do come from inside, and when I have been upset before when Frank has said, "Why don't you get a job?" it's because I felt like a victim. I didn't feel that it was anything that I was doing for myself but that I was a victim. Now, I think I am incapable of being victimized. The only person that can victimize me is myself. It may turn out in the end that I don't really think the PhD program is worth all the trouble. I don't think I'd have any trouble getting into the Jungian training program. It may be that by reading some of the books the Jung Foundation publishes, I'll get more out of it. I also called the National Organization for Women and the Women's Liberation Movement in this area. I was told about a bookshop that's not too far away from the discount bookshop on Connecticut Avenue, which has an excellent collection of books on women. I think the next time I have my haircut, I'll go there. I was thinking that the next time I go to Dr. Kuhn's or to Carol Ann's, I want to plan my day and either have lunch with Roselle and Shirley or go to the library or bookstore for the day. In fact, I've been toying with the idea of going to New York on December 2. I think Anna is going there to hear a talk on the psychological aspects of the Women's Movement given by a Jungian analyst, and I think it would be great to go too. I'd also like to go to the library at the Jung Foundation. There is also a picture collection there called ARAS (Archive for Research in Archetypal Symbolism). I would also like to go to the Feminist Repertory Theatre in New York. I have been thinking about that. I don't know what arrangements I would make for the children, but maybe, I could work something out. Maybe, I could persuade Anna to come down from New York and spend a few days here. But I do want to do more recordings. I have so many things that I want to say. I suppose Connie would say that it's all therapy, and I suppose that it is. But that too is worthwhile.

Thinking about all these things really zaps my mind: thinking about the new clothes I'm going to buy, thinking about writing, and about these two programs. It turns out that the universities in this area do offer courses in women's studies. It would be interesting to take one of them. I shouldn't be tempted to squander my energies riding around to different things, but it might be fun to call these universities and to find out more about, for instance, taking a writing course. I've got so much to write, I don't have time to stop and take a course, and that's the way I feel. Everything seems so incredibly and intensely exciting. I think that not only do I not want to squander my energies, but I want to be careful that I do what I want to do and not get sidetracked into spending a lot of time writing letters to people that I'm not that keen on writing to in the first place.

I've been thinking about ordering Christmas cards, and I've been thinking about Christmas gifts. I think that I might give people UNICEF calendars as gifts. It looks to me like a nice gift, and I think it would be a worthwhile gift for people whether or not they have children.

Yesterday, we got a little gift in the mail from Zoe, a birthday present for Katherine Louise. It was the most adorable little book from Rand McNally. I have seen so many of those books, but I've never seen one as cute as this. In fact, most of them are not nearly as nice as this one. Zoe is so thoughtful. She is a beautiful person.

So many of the things that Jill Morton said about New York brought back the whole New York experience to me. Jill said that, for instance, people in New York will say, "Well, have you seen such-and-such movie? You haven't? Why not?" Being current on things is a kind of mad passion. First, it was civil rights. Then it was the war in Vietnam. Then it was Women's Liberation, and now, it's drugs. So everyone is doing something for drug rehabilitation. Everyone is so au courant. There is no past and no future, and she calls it a lack of roots. She said she didn't like a place that was like Sleepy Hollow. On the other hand, there seems to be something wrong with the life in New York. Everybody there is so conscious, so rational, and it does seem that you are all in one shared area. Even Cambridge and Boston have slight variations, and there is variation in lifestyle as well. New York is probably more conformist.

Jill said she had given a dinner party, and one of the women at the dinner party said about her banana soufflé dessert, "What! You're having bananas after what was done in the Dominican Republic?" Everything is so completely and totally political that there is no act that is not political. It seemed that way to me too. It wasn't so much that it seemed political, but it seemed that everybody was really on the qui vive and on the surface, perpetually distracted from anything very deep. Yet the Jung Foundation is there, as well as the headquarters for the Women's Movement. The whole Women's Movement is centered in New York.

At any rate, it just brought back to me how I felt when I worked there at the New York Public Library and when I started at Columbia University. I remember especially when I was working at the Yorkville branch of the New York Public Library. In fact, I tried to write a story about my colleague Jim Robertson because he was the only person that didn't seem like New York to me. Jim and I used to talk about the ocean. I tried to write a story about how he represented the ocean to me, a slower way of life in Boston, a kind of adolescence, a certain dreaminess. Several times, I've thought about writing that story about cleaning my room and about the pencil. I should get them out and work on them even though I was put off by Connie's response to them. She said they weren't really "fictional enough." It was strange to hear Jill talk about New York because she characterized a response that I had had myself exactly.

Yesterday, after writing how euphoric I felt and how I felt that this was what I would have wished my first pregnancy to be if I had known what to wish for and how it seemed like a combination of a pregnancy and a honeymoon, I had a strange experience. Last night, Frank called me at about 7:00 p.m. and said he was going to be late. He hadn't come home for lunch, and he got home at around 8:30 p.m. from work. Both the children were still up, although they were in their pajamas and ready to go to bed. Thomas had had no nap, and both children seemed very tired. Thomas seemed as though he were coming down with a cold. I had Frank's dinner in the warming oven, and for about two hours before that, I had been half-waiting for him to come home. Every imaginable thing that Katherine Louise could have gotten into, she got into. The kids dumped all their toys out everywhere and pulled all kinds of stuff out of the bureau drawers in their room. I kept pulling her out of the bathrooms until I finally locked the doors. She was either playing in the toilet or dropping things in the toilet or climbing in the sink in my bathroom or trying to get the razor blades out of the medicine chest, and Thomas hit her several times. She fell down another time. The kids pulled all the books off the bookshelves. By the time Frank came home, I felt that staying sane was really an effort. I felt utterly exhausted, and Thomas wanted a raisin sandwich, and it seemed that the last lap of getting him into bed was unbelievable. He wanted Frank to read to him. Finally, he got into bed, and I stretched out on the couch. I know there's litter everywhere. I feel as though I'm going to suffocate with the kids' toys and the kids' clothes and stuff thrown all around. I feel as though I can't even move. I thought, "Well, I really should go to bed. I am that tired." I said to Frank, "I think I'll go to bed. I feel awfully tired." And he said, "You're kidding, you're not tired, are you?" I stayed there in a state of torpor.

We started talking about B. F. Skinner and the article in *Time* magazine about him. Frank said it was strange that Skinner himself didn't go to live in a commune but that probably, it was because of his wife. Probably, his wife didn't like free sex. It was a complete projection. I don't feel that I have to feel personally attacked if people attack wives, but he was coming to conclusions, left and right. He said that his old boss, Corat, hated his wife and would have murdered her if he could have gotten away with it and that wives really don't give you any goodies—or if they do, they make you pay a fantastically high price for the goodies—and that wives make you work and that you have to work all the time. "You know, it's really just killing," he said, and he went on and on and on. I can't help but feel that if he feels this as a generalization, he must feel that it applies to me somewhat or, at least, that it applies to the institution of wifedom. I was tempted to say, "Do you think this applies to us?" It makes me feel that I don't want to be his wife anymore. It is so horrible to be a wife. I have always felt that he has cloaked me in the robe of an authority figure, and he has a number of assumptions, such as women want marriage and men don't, that all women are always pushing for marriage, and that they make you work all the time. I do think that this is true in some cases, but I don't think that it is, by any means, true in all cases, and I wouldn't like to think that it was true in our case. I would like to have a loving relationship with Frank. I would like to have a fantastic man-woman relationship. But there is something horrible about the institution of marriage. There is something degrading about it, and I have to constantly remind myself that I am a person and that I am separate from this institution and that I have to think of myself as a person and only legally or minimally a wife. Then he got up, and I asked him to turn off the oven. The oven was turned to warm, and I said, "Would you turn off the oven?" He said, "What the hell is the oven on for?" Finally, he said, "I must sound grouchy." The strange thing is that he had told me how he wasn't tired at all and how great he felt because he had hypnotized himself at lunch time, but it was as though he was telling me, in this not-too-indirect way, that men really do hate women. There wasn't any way I could confront him or grapple with it, but I felt my gorge rising. I was irritated at a very basic level. Then he said that if my leg was bothering me, he would hypnotize me, which he did do. Then I said that I did feel more relaxed from my waist up, but I also had this other strange feeling in my other leg, similar to the touch of arthritis that I had when I was pregnant with Katherine. It hurt to put weight on my leg. It felt like my hip joint socket was dry. Frank said to me, "I guess you really want to have that pain in your leg." I felt so tired. I couldn't think fast enough of any way to confront him with this, and he was saying things like "Do you think Alfred would marry Hetty now if he met her walking down the street?" He said that he thought none of the men would marry their wives. He has said many things like this before. It is too horrible to be a wife. I felt afterward that I wanted to wash all the ickiness off, that this is too degrading to be part of, and that marriage is quite different from a loving relationship, and I felt that, in all honesty, I couldn't be a wife. As time wore on, his spirit just rose and rose. I felt as though I shouldn't stay up without a snack or some coffee. I asked him if he wanted anything. No, he didn't want anything. He didn't want to gain weight. He was talking to me about hypnotism and how great it was and how fabulous it was. Finally, it was about 12:30 a.m., and I said, "If you met me, would you marry me now?" He said, "Well, you know, if you used some of your tools." I guess I was asking for it to say anything at all to him. I have the strangest feeling as though I were done violence to in my role as wife. I felt disconcerted.

It was about twelve minutes before one. In view of the fact that I am pregnant, hadn't had any kind of nap, have two youngsters to take care of, had a stupid cough, and had to have a chest x-ray, and his attitude was "Gee, you're kidding me, you're tired?" I began to feel nauseated. I had eaten my dinner at about 7:00 p.m. By about 1:00 a.m., I began to feel woozy. Frank did get me some ginger ale. We went into the bedroom, and he was in a very amorous mood. I felt absolutely and completely furious. First of all, he had heaped insults upon insults on wives and women. Finally, we sat out here for so long, and he waited until 1:00 a.m. to make his amorous advances. By that time, I was just about in a state of collapse. It was as though he were teasing me and rejecting me. And then, of course, he could sleep the following morning. Not only did I have to get up with the children, but I would probably have been woken up during the night by them as well. Sure enough, we went to bed at about 1:00 a.m., and at about 5:30 a.m., Katherine started to cry—she wanted a bottle. I woke up, and the rest of this whole experience was fresh in my mind. After I put her into bed with her bottle, I could not go back to sleep. I thought, maybe,

I should get up and record how I felt, or maybe, I should tell Frank when he woke up. I thought that he was inconsiderate, and I feel as though he is not aware of me. I am trying to communicate with a mechanism that is much cruder. I felt that not once had he really talked to me. I thought that if I said anything to him in the first place, it's always a delayed reaction to something I have always been accused of, like waiting two weeks and then telling somebody how upset I was about something they said. Also, I know it would be unpleasant to start telling him something because I felt that I had rubbed him the wrong way, and he just never knew the difference. And then I started thinking that there wasn't much point in saying anything unless I say it much, much earlier. Say it right then and there on the spot, and don't let it slide by, but I was so tired last night that I couldn't even get off the couch to go to bed Before that, I had started thinking that I didn't want to be a wife. I don't want to take anything from anybody. I don't want to be supported by somebody. I want to support myself. I want to walk around at least with pride that I can support myself.

Then I began to think that instead of spending time on that, why don't I go to New York for that talk on December 2? Why don't I buy a Tano handbag? I decided, "I know what I'll do. I'll order that Beldoch Popper slack suit and wait on the dress because the dress is not buttoned down the front, and I wouldn't wear it much in the winter." I should go through some of the *New York Times* to see if they have any other ads for things that I like better than the ones I found. I'll try to get a Tano handbag and some nice underwear, and I'll find out about the training for Jungian analysts. I would give anything to have some time for myself. I feel that right now, I could write and write and write nonstop; I have so many things to say. There is an impersonal quality that one craves, a time for one's own personal emotions.

It was strange that one of the nights that we were on vacation, *The Pumpkin Eater*, with Anne Bancroft, was shown on television, and I saw a little of it. This woman's predicament was understandable; she only felt complete when she was pregnant, but her husband persuaded her to get sterilized. Her own sense of sexual identity was dependent upon her being fertile so that there was no alternative for her except to completely crack up, having such a strong drive in one direction and then having her husband persuade her to destroy this drive. Aside from what her predicament was and what happened, I realize that when a person is completely mired in emotions like that, it's like being lost in a jungle. He might as well wave goodbye to you.

I was thinking of getting up in the morning and telling Frank what he said, but I know he would only be extremely defensive, and it would all end up worse. It's as though I want to sing a song, and the song is "I Am

Beautiful although I Am a Wife, I Am Beautiful although I Am a Wife,"
and "I Am a Person," and "I Am," and the wife part is really infinitesimal.
It was so strange to wake up at five-thirty in the morning. I felt as though
I should wake Frank up, especially since he felt so great; he should get up
and take care of the baby because when I told him I was tired, he said,
"You're kidding." He can sleep all morning when I have to get up with the
kids. It seems so unfair, so truly unfair.

This morning, we woke up, and we made love. When I'm not exhausted
to the point of falling over, I have such a strong sexual desire for Frank,
and he can make me feel so great that way. I could love him just for that;
the physical contact with him is so exquisite. But last night, I was so upset
by what he said that I couldn't respond to him in that way. I guess that if
you hate somebody, it is difficult to make love with that person.

Frank said a strange thing earlier at dinner. He said, in connection with
hypnosis, that he wouldn't mind having a little analysis himself because
he has quirks in his nature. For example, he absolutely will not go into a
barbershop. The past few times he went into a barbershop, which was a few
years ago, he was draped and sat up there like a fool with people looking
at him only to have someone give him a horrible haircut. It's difficult for
him to go into a new social setting too, to go to a party with a lot of strange
people. He mentioned his mother and that he felt some of the same social
uneasiness she apparently felt. He feels the same way about classes and
schools and structured situations. He is very grateful for what he got out
of them, and when he goes to a meeting of some kind, he feels exhilarated
and stimulated. But initially, he just can't stand it. I know that this is true,
and I think that it is a reaction to his parents, and it's a reaction against any
setting that has any kind of structure to it or any sort of formality, where
there is even the slightest rule or regulation. He feels as though it's a terrible
imposition, to the point where he is incapable of making anything final
by himself or capable of delegating anything. He sets up some situations
where I have to ask him for things on the shopping lists. He either loses
the shopping list or he goes to the store but doesn't look at it because he
doesn't get what is on the list. He does very well as far as the shopping goes.
He brings home plenty of steaks and good food, but he doesn't get what is
on the list, and many times, I have to write something down twenty times
before he gets it. It's as though he is begging me to nag him. It's both like
repulsion and attraction to this kind of system, where he's got to have an
external force. He's got to have the thing really pushing him. He claims he
would like a situation where in order to have his lunch, he would have to go
out and catch the fish or go out and pull the vegetables from the garden.
He likes the pressure that's absolutely now as though you are standing there
waiting for him to go to the store and get the toilet paper. He has to have

that urgent pressure right then and there. He never delegates anything to me, and he never sets up a system such as "Give me shopping lists on this day and this day." But he mentioned himself that he wouldn't mind having some kind of analysis because of this. He mentioned that earlier at dinner time, but I didn't say anything because I don't want to hurt his feelings. But I mentioned Dr. Clark, our former pediatrician, to him, and I mentioned to him that I think people pave their own way to failure, that I thought Dr. Clark was a good example of somebody who could probably be tremendously successful, but he didn't want to be. He has failure so built into himself that he could never succeed. The result was such a weird evening because he was making me furious because he was being aggressive toward me. On the other hand, I thought, "Is there something wrong with me?" He did do a few nice things. He got some ginger ale for me, and he tried to hypnotize me. He does try to do nice things for me. But it was so weird. It was like one of those experiences in a Bergman movie where the reality that he is in and the reality I am in are just so different. You feel so close to the person, and yet you feel so far away. My mind was galloping, thinking about what to get for Christmas presents, and I was thinking that Thomas needed some new clothes for school and that it would be great to get the kids a record player for Christmas. When I'm feeding the baby, that would be a good time to play records. I was thinking about clothes that I wanted to buy and things that I wanted to do, and I decided that instead of dwelling on the incident last night, it is better to have my own goals that I can work toward. I don't know whether you would call it a tempest in a teapot or a microcosm in the living room, but it seems like a fantastic drama. I do think that I should try to respond at the moment, and that's the only thing to do.

Katherine is awake from her nap. This is the kind of experience I used to find terrifying. I would be in a situation where there are no markers and no guidelines. It seems as though it would be possible for two people to destroy each other, and then I began to think that there are so many things I want to do for the children. It's not worth spending time on some of this, except right there on the spot at the moment. It's bound to come up again. It's come up before, and it's bound to come up again. I should not lose sight of my own goals and my own ideas of myself and what I can do. Maybe, I'm paranoid about certain things, or maybe, I am unduly sensitive to some of the things Frank says. I don't want to start telling him that he shouldn't say this or he shouldn't say that. He should feel absolutely free to say what he wants to say. Maybe, I have an exalted idea of what I am capable of doing, but I do feel as though I can do anything.

Thursday, October 14, 1971

One of my most pressing needs is time to myself, and I suppose it must have a cumulative effect. Two or three days without any time to myself is excruciating. It feels as though I am squeezed into a smaller and smaller box until after a while, I am going to lash out.

I have entered the last trimester of the pregnancy; I have noticed a change—I feel heavier, less able to navigate easily. My need for time to myself is more acute now than at other times. If I had more time, I know exactly what I'd do. I feel drawn in two directions and more strongly in one of the two. I have a desire to do more things; I'm sorting out, preparing, and anticipating—thinking about what I'm going to do for Christmas, for example.

There's also a greater dreaminess at the same time. I can remember when I was pregnant with Katherine Louise, I found myself constantly cleaning out bureau drawers and going through my closets and dealing with notebooks and papers and letters that I had accumulated. It is somewhat the same this time, but in a way, it's more creative. I want to keep this diary, and I also want to go on with the typing. In fact, I called Mrs. Fisk. She had a baby boy last October 2 and named him Shayne Michael. I asked her if she would do the typing for the whole project when she felt up to it. I have also been thinking about what I want to do after I get this typing done. I'll have this pregnancy diary on tape, but what do I want to do after that? I want to do a postscript on motherhood, and also, there are two or three other things that I would like to do. Then I began to think that I had kept a diary most of the time, and when I try to do other writings, I have to get the diary writing out of the way. I've been thinking about this recently, and

I thought I want to keep the pregnancy diary, but at the same time, I would like to work on something else. I felt that I really should get my notebooks and some of my notes in order. It seems that I could boil some of this writing down so that I have four to six projects that I could work on, all of them at the same time, or I could work on them successively. I have found that very exciting, and as soon as I'm finished checking for corrections the typing that Mrs. Fisk has already done, I'm going to go through some of my notes and sort them out and go through some of my notebooks and try to line up perhaps four things that I'd like to do. Maybe, the tape machine will enable me to work on more than one thing at a time. It would be interesting to both tape and write at the same time. I would like to know what Anna and Connie think of what I've written. I think it's too watered down to be anything good, and that's one of the things about the tape machine. One has to talk at such a fast rate that everything is diluted; whereas when you write, it can be more condensed, pithier. As a result, what I say sounds trite, sentimental, clichéd, and, in general, too watered down. It all needs to be condensed and abstracted. I'll have to see the whole thing before I know exactly what I want to do. I don't really have any clear ideas about what I would like to do with it. I have been going through it. I keep thinking about all of these things that I would like to do, and if I weren't pregnant, I wouldn't feel that way to such an extent. I would give anything if there were any way to get a few days when I could get up in the morning and work on this. I would give anything, but I have so little time.

Today, Thomas went to school at 1:00 p.m., and Frank went to work. I put Katherine down for her nap, and she never went to sleep. I was all set up to do some recording. I felt I had to do some. No sooner had I gotten the tape machine plugged in than one of the workmen, the man who belongs to a barbershop quartet, came. He talks, talks, talks about his barbershop quartet and the shows that they put on and what a good time they've had and that his wife is in the quartet. He refers to their friends in terms of whether the woman is a soprano or whether the man is a tenor or a baritone. All the time that he is talking, he wants you to stroke his ego. I just can't stand him. But to see him coming up across the lawn while I am waiting for Katherine to go to sleep, I think if I see one more person like that, I am going to scream. He had the World Series blaring on the radio in his truck and sat out front listening to it for such a long time before he even came up to the door.

Katherine seems to sleep so little. When she takes a nap, it's only for a couple of hours, and often, I don't get her to sleep until two, and at three, I have to pick Thomas up from school, and I don't seem to be able to get her to sleep before ten-thirty at night. I put both children into bed; Thomas goes to sleep, and she stands up in her crib and cries. I get her up, I put her back, I get her up, I put her back—I do this maybe three times before she finally settles down. Because she took no nap today, she has gone into bed early, but it seems fantastic to work from eight in the morning until eleven at night, every day, seven days a week.

Yesterday was Wednesday. At breakfast time, I was sitting at the table, thinking that it is inhuman for housewives not to have a day off, for mothers of small children not to have a day off. Eventually, it must begin to interfere with the mothering not to have a day off. Every mother of small children should have two eight-hour days off a week to pursue her interests and restore herself. Unless the children sleep a great deal, it's impossible to do this. Sometimes, one is so consistently and repeatedly interrupted that it is fantastically frustrating. I was sitting at the table thinking that, and I wondered how it was in times gone by when you didn't have days off. Living was so different. It is only with this kind of suburban life and life in a development in the nuclear family where one is virtually locked up with the kids. It's not just that. It's not like being locked up with them in the Louvre or somewhere interesting, somewhere that is naturally beautiful where the kids can run. There's even no place where you can put them in a baby carriage and walk them to where there is activity so that they are distracted. There are no closed-in yards, and these houses are so small, at least ours is so small, that there are no separate playrooms for the children. The people here are so nuclear-family oriented that there is never anyone around who would give the child attention or read the child a story for fifteen minutes so that the mother could shower and dress. This isolated lifestyle, probably, is worse than any previous ones. There are no extended family present to give time to the children.

Yesterday, I had a dream. It was a dream about Denise Silverman. She called me and said she was in town, and I went to see her. She was in an apartment, somewhere like the Watergate. Her circumstances were similar to Jill Morton's. She was there by herself. Her plans seemed a little vague. She was going to Atlantic City and then to some other places. She seemed exuberant and happy. She said that David was hemping it, and I said, "You mean marijuana?" and she said, "Yeah." I think she had the children with her, but they were completely out of sight. When I left and we walked down the corridor toward the elevator, she met two or three people and she said of one, "Oh, that person works for the governor." Then this other woman said to her, "Did Ann do your eyebrows?" Denise said yes. Then the woman said, "I thought so. They look so lovely." She had somebody to do her eyebrows and somebody to do her nails and somebody to do her hair. Everything that she talked about reflected money or concern for money. So when I left there, I sensed that Denise, like Jill, was having some sort of crisis in her marriage, but I never pointedly asked, and she didn't go into it very much. When I left there, I felt poor. It's like the time when Jill was here and, at the table, said, "Gee, wouldn't it be great to have money?" I said, "It's strange, but I never felt that way." I had always felt that the lack of money never kept me from doing anything I wanted to do. I guess I'm a perfect poor man's wife. I realized afterward how stupid that sounded. I asked Jill what she would do if she had money, and she said, "Well, it would be so nice not to have to worry about it. It would be fun to spend the summers in Europe." And of course, Frank agreed that this would be great. There would be so many things that one could do. Afterward, I was thinking that I must have sounded silly to say what I said.

In some ways, this dream had to do with that conversation about money because it stuck in my mind, and I have said the same thing to one or two other people. Finally, I decided that I'm not going to say that anymore because it sounds too absurd, and when I stop and think about it, it was true in my life before I got married that I always felt I had enough money to do anything I wanted to do. Maybe, I lack the imagination to spend money, but since Thomas was born, I feel that we are far less able to do things I'd like to do, and if I had money, even a little money, I would at least have a cleaning lady and a babysitter every now and then. I certainly would get the typing done, and I wouldn't worry about it so much. I would probably have Carol Ann do my haircuts more often, and I would probably have a few more clothes.

Returning to the dream: when I left, I felt poor. My clothes are so shabby, and the house is so shabby. It was very peculiar. I either continued to dream or I woke up and then consciously thought of this. I suddenly thought that I don't feel poor because what I want to do is something else. I want to record a lot of things, and to write, and I don't care about personal possessions and material objects. It's such a strange paradox; I feel more motivated to write than ever before, and I have less time than ever before. I have almost no time. If I had a little more money, I would make a few more long-distance calls to Boston, and I would even go up there, so probably, it's not completely true that I wouldn't do anything differently, but basically, what I really want to do is create and give, so it is still true that I feel that way.

A week ago, Saturday, I got a letter from Toni Yeats and a collection of her poems that were written in English. She also sent a leaf, a red-and-yellow leaf from Vermont. Toni said, "To Katherine, whose eyes are full of wonder at life," and then in the letter, she said how happy they were to see us and how I seemed to be surrounded by an atmosphere of life. Anyway, I read the poems, and they are fantastic, especially considering that she has written them in English. They truly are fantastic. I cried when I read them. They are so beautiful! She is able to be authentic and create images for the way she sees things. I think that is something worth doing, not just having a lot of money; there is a fantastic number of things that you can do that would be a waste of time—like, to some extent shopping and traveling. These are things that people with money do, and one can waste a lot of time doing these things.

I was so excited about the poems that I showed them to Frank when he first came home, and then a couple of hours later, I said, "Oh, did you see the poems?" He said, "No, I just got in here." He gave me a defensive explanation—how he just got in and how he only now had a chance to sit down. But he did look at the poems while he was eating, and Thomas wanted the leaf, so Frank gave the leaf to Thomas and not just to admire it. He gave it to him, and I was furious that he did that. I had given Thomas the leaf earlier in the day for him to look at, and he was just holding it between his thumb and his forefinger and twirling it back and forth, back and forth, looking at it. I was absolutely furious, and I took the leaf away from Thomas. Thomas cried bitterly. He was absolutely heartbroken. Nevertheless, I took the leaf from him. I was trying to get dinner. Katherine was extremely fussy and down deep; I had been annoyed with Frank when I said to him so enthusiastically, "Did you see Toni's letter and the poems?" And then when he gave the leaf to Thomas, I thought that it was going to get crushed or torn, and I took the leaf away from Thomas. He cried brokenheartedly, and about five or ten minutes after that, Thomas was asleep, leaning against Frank. He had had no nap. This must have been 7:30 p.m. We carried him into bed. He woke up half an hour after that, fussy and crying.

By this time, I had begun to feel bad about having taken the leaf away from Thomas. What is a leaf? Not only just what is a leaf, but really isn't it nicer for him to have some appreciation of it even if the leaf gets ripped up than to save it for posterity? What good is it going to do where it is now? I had put it away in a bookcase. There was drama surrounding that leaf that Toni had sent.

Frank and I were talking the other day about the women we know who had remarried and who have all married very wealthy men. One woman has married a relative of Rockefeller's, and he owns a house in England, one in Ireland, and a couple in the United States. Another woman I know married a man who is very successful in business. He flies his own airplane. They live in Cheverly. The third one is married to somebody who is a representative in the Washington area for a large oil company. He is a lobbyist. These women are about forty years old. Marriage is their way of life, and they are going to succeed and progress up the ladder within this particular framework. For the woman whose career is marriage, her attitude toward marriage is the same toward it as if law or medicine were her career. One doesn't want to progress backward.

When I was sitting at the breakfast table on Wednesday morning, thinking that it's too hard not to ever have a day off, it seemed to me as though nobody takes it easier than Frank. I would say that he is one of the most leisurely people I have ever met, and he wouldn't hurry for anybody. You couldn't get him to hurry no matter what. The work he does is unbelievable. It is to his credit that he can make as much money as he does on the number of hours that he works. I said to him, "Every time I talk to women around Kettering, they ask me, 'When is your husband's house office going to open?'" I've told him several times, "I think you would find it worthwhile to go ahead and open the dental office here because I think that the women here would be extremely conscientious mothers." Frank's reply is "Well, I'm not really a sixty-hour-a-week man." He has his guard up all the time about working more than he is working, and if I say to him, "Frank, I work about ninety hours a week," he'll say, "That's not work, that's fulfillment." He makes a mockery of anything I say to him like that. He says it and just passes it off. I don't think he thinks about it particularly. It makes me furious. If I were to say something, I guess I would probably say something terribly mean.

Anyway, I was just sitting there thinking about how I put the children to bed at night. It's one thing to finally get Katherine Louise asleep by 10:30 or 11:00 p.m., and then invariably, I'll sit up for about an hour, and then I'll say to Frank, "I think I'll go to bed." And he'll say, "You're not tired, are you?" That makes me furious. I don't know why, but it does. I am the one who gets up during the night to tend to the children. A couple of times, he has gotten up for them, but it seems that they don't go back to sleep for him. Frank can take care of Thomas pretty well. While I'm sitting here at the table, my arms are aching. I feel that I've held them up over my head all night after I've been up with the children. I want to get all the dishes done. I have laundry to do downstairs. I want to get the kids dressed. I made a pound cake. I didn't have any time off Monday night, and Monday is supposed to be my night off. Frank always gets home from work about 8:30 or 9:00 p.m. That is the night he takes to go to the bank and do other errands. I think he should work whatever number of hours that he wants to, but he is so defensive about even a suggestion that he work a little more. On the other hand, he is always saying to me that I should get a job, that what I do here isn't work but fulfillment, or "You're not tired, are you?" Around midmorning, after I had gotten the children dressed, I sat down, and he said to me, "Meditating?" That hurt me. It's similar to my Monday night off. He tells me that he is going to give me Monday night off, but I never get Monday night off. It's the same thing with my allowance. I'm supposed to get a weekly allowance, but I never get it. I think it's been a year since I've seen my last allowance. And then there's the way he reacted to the typing, and at some point, he told me he would get up with the kids one morning. I said, "Well, if you want me to, I'll get up with them. If you take them out for me, that's the big thing. If you'd only take them out for a walk in the morning, then I wouldn't have to stand on my feet so much." He said he would do that, but he has never done it. One morning, I wanted to take a shower, so I asked him if he would watch the kids just for a few minutes while I got ready, and he said, "Well, sort of, but I have to work on the car. I'll watch them the best I can." It's a no and a yes answer. He went out, and I sat down in the chair by the window. Thomas and Katherine went into Mrs. Real's house. I sat there and sat there and sat there because little Katherine cannot go over the Real's front concrete steps. She's already fallen there once. I didn't feel as though I could go into the shower. Finally, I put on a dress so I could go out and watch them. Frank came in and said, "What's the matter? Are you sick?" I said, "No, but I thought you would watch the children for me." And he said, "Well, I've got to fix the car. I'm fixing it for you because otherwise, you'll have to walk everywhere." I took the children out to the playground, but the whole time I was there, I felt like crying.

When I came back, I got lunch. I told Frank lunch was ready, and in the wake of it, Katherine was into everything. Frank took forever to come to the table. Later, I asked him to carry the laundry basket downstairs. He waited four days before he did it. I asked him to get me some stamps. I never did get the stamps. I find all of this demeaning. It seems pointless to tell him how I feel because he gets so defensive. I think he is very resentful of me. I think he thinks that I'm not working. He feels terribly sorry for himself because he has to work as if he's working all the time for me. When he asked me, "Meditating?" I suppose he could have meant it in an offhand way, but it made me feel that I hated him, just hated him. I have horrible feelings, and I find it hard to deal with feelings of hate, repulsion, and aversion. Afterward, I don't like myself. I do want to feel loving and giving, and I do want to give a lot to the children. A person can use up a lot of energy in hate. I should try to give love as much as I possibly can. I do want to be a giver.

Frank's view of me and my view of myself are so different. After a while, I begin to think about how I can defend myself. But I don't want to spend a lot of energy on that. When you're not married, your feelings of dissatisfaction are directed toward yourself. When you are married, you have somebody you can dump these feelings on. I felt so much that way yesterday. It seems he doesn't like me, or he thinks I'm just a freeloader here.

I did call Mrs. Fisk yesterday, and I am going to have her do all the typing. My first response is to think I don't want to take anything from him. These things are always cumulative. It probably had something to do with the dream I had and feeling so poor and also something to do with sitting at the breakfast table thinking to myself that I never got that time off in the morning that he said he was going to give me. I never get my Monday night off. How can you be pleasant and cheerful when you work seven days a week from eight in the morning until eleven at night? How can you seem enthusiastic and energetic when your sleep is disturbed once or twice every night? The person that you try to tell about how you feel tells you that you're not really working, you're finding fulfillment. Then at the slightest suggestion that he do something, he's not about to do it. I think it's obvious that he doesn't live in a town because it seems too hierarchical and there are too many authority figures around. He would be too well-known. He can be anonymous in our present setting. I think he is hesitant about putting the office downstairs because he's afraid he might have to work harder. What's awful is this feeling that I get when I don't really want to engage with him. After a while, it's defeating.

I think of Helen's sister, Dottie, and how she berated the man that she was married to for decades. She was married for forty years and finally got divorced. Apparently, she is very depressed now. I can see why she is depressed—she spent her life hating this man.

It was a combination of the dream about Denise and then feeling so poor in that dream and then sitting at the table and thinking that there is no such thing for me as a day off. This must change. It's an unbelievable setup. It's excruciating after a while—it is a cumulative hardship not to have any time to oneself. I suppose some of the things that I have been criticized for are true. I don't respond until I'm terribly crowded. There probably is a wall around me, and I'm living behind that wall, and as long as nothing impinges too hard on the wall, anything that goes on outside the wall is okay. But when there is too much pressure on the wall and it is pushed too hard, I begin to react. When I don't have any time to myself for several days running, I'm ready to tear my hair out. It is true. I need a little time to myself every day. I don't know why.

A couple of weeks ago, we saw a car crash. Two cars collided on Enterprise Road, and for days afterward, Thomas played this game where he would ride the tyke bike and then fall off and call, "Sissy, get me up, get me up, get me up." He was playing dead. He also did a lot of drawings of car crashes.

It seems strange that now, I have more drive to write than ever before, and it's more difficult to get any time to do it. I feel so motivated to do a lot of different things. As far as Frank is concerned, I always say to myself the only thing to do is to respond at the moment. Don't let the things he says hurt and then build up feelings about it. Respond at the moment, at the moment, at the moment.

Friday, November 5, 1971

I have not done any recording since October 14. The past three weeks have been so busy that I just haven't had a chance. They have been an amazing three weeks in many ways.

For some reason, after I got back from vacation, I was thinking a lot about the motherhood work, mostly because I had given copies of it to Connie and Anna. I began to wonder a lot about what they thought of it. I had all kinds of qualms about having given it to them. I thought, maybe, I seemed too critical of Frank. I could well imagine that Connie would be angry. I kept thinking about it and thinking about it. What did I really say? Until I did that tape on motherhood, the whole experience was so close to me. All the day-by-day horrors were so close to me, and yet once I did it, it seemed to get farther and farther away because now, I don't feel the same way about Frank that I felt when I did that. There's been so much happiness since then. The experience did get farther away. It was strange to think that I did, at one time, feel that way, but I don't feel that way now, and I thought, "Well, what did I say?" I was wondering about the tape partly because of that and partly because of listening to the second big tape on the small cassettes. They were taped just before we went on vacation, and I hadn't listened to them before, and I wanted to listen to them before having them typed. Then the thought occurred to me that I could send the typed manuscript of the motherhood tapes to the magazine *AFRA*. All of a sudden, it occurred to me. When I realized the possibilities of what that meant in terms of typing, I was very pleased because I thought that paying to have the motherhood tapes typed was almost too much to ask of Frank in terms of money, when he should probably spend the money on his office. Then I thought, "Why just have that one thing taped and never do anything else?" Fantastic doors started opening very fast, and in one flash, I saw the possibilities of sending that work to *AFRA*. I realized that I could have the rest of the motherhood tapes typed and then anything else that I wanted typed. I began to think that at some point, I would have the pregnancy diary typed. I have some of the preliminary motherhood tapes typed, the ones that I did in September and October of 1968. Suddenly, it seemed that typing was a real possibility, that it wasn't a problem, and that I had figured out a way it could be done. I suddenly had the technology, and I was so excited about this that I had another, I don't know what you'd call it, insight or vision, partly going over the corrections on the typed manuscript before getting it ready to send to *AFRA*, thinking about it so much because I had given copies to Connie and Anna, listening to reel two of the cassettes, keeping a notebook of postscripts to the motherhood tapes—it all began to proliferate.

I began to think that I wanted to do something else besides keeping a diary. Before I was married, whenever I did any writing, it seemed that I had to write to get a lot of things out of the way and off my chest, to clear the way for something else, and what usually happened was that by the time I finished writing in the diary, it was time to go out, go to work, or do something that had to be done. It seems to me, in a way, faster to tape it than to write it, so I began to think it would be possible to work on something else in addition to the pregnancy diary. One morning, just as I was waking up, I thought, "What do I want to do then? What should I do next?" I had ideas here and there for this and that. All of a sudden, I thought, "Why don't I go through my notes and go through some of the things I've already started, see if I can organize them into some shape, and start working on them one by one? And maybe, it will be possible to tape some of them. Maybe, it would be possible to adapt that material to tape." It was as though I had a vision of all the writing that I wanted to do. I thought of a couple of stories that had something to do with my early childhood and some of the family things that I wanted to do and then some of the things from later on in my life. It was an utterly amazing experience. I had never had anything happen quite like that before. I saw very clearly what I wanted to do. So from about October 14 onward, I went through my notebooks. I just looked at the notebooks to see what they were, and I arranged them. I separated the diaries from the things that I had attempted to write, and I put the diaries in chronological order, and the other works that I did I tried to arrange into some order. It seemed that things were proliferating at a faster and faster rate. While I was going through the notebooks, I decided I would take my notes and put them into folders and then work on the folders. I was working on this like mad.

I had also been thinking about library school because Frank had asked me why I didn't get a PhD in library science. I called the University of Maryland to find out whether I would have to take the graduate record exams and whether I would get any credit for the masters degree that I already have. I thought I would look into it to see what was involved because Frank had suggested it to me as a good idea. The other thing was that I was toying with the idea of Jungian analysis. I don't know that much about it. I thought I might try to find out whether it would be possible to commute to New York and whether it would be possible to do this with the educational background that I have. I'm still not sure whether it would be possible. I believe that everything is possible if you really want to do it. There is one person listed in this area who is a Jungian analyst. She lives in Chevy Chase, and I think I might call her. I feel that if I do either one of these things, I also would continue with my taping. I also feel, and I know this is because of the pregnancy more than anything else, fantastically creative. If I could only work on some of this.

I know that after the baby is born, I'll be fantastically busy. As it is, I'm very busy. I wish I had more time. I feel I'm on borrowed time now. After January, after the baby is born, everything will be different. Right now, there are sad times, but it's almost as though I'm on a permanent high. I'm going pell-mell, and pell-mell on borrowed time.

It's the time of year when the light has changed so much and the leaves are so pretty. I like this time of year better than any other. I feel great. I know that this will be my last pregnancy, and I feel so dreamy. I say "creative" when I probably should say "dreamy." But it does make me feel like moving into myself somewhat, and I wonder if I'm giving enough to the children.

It was strange to go through some of those notes and see the kinds of things that I had been occupied with. I can see such a fantastic progression and relationship in the earlier and later things and how they connect with each other. The problem of form doesn't matter so much. This has been liberating. I feel so fantastically motivated. Life is incredibly exciting. There never is enough time. Certainly, there never is enough time to oneself, and I have been reading through the diaries, and it's really strange that sometimes, when I'm feeling hurt or overworked or out of sorts with Frank or with myself, I rail against my life. Yet when I look back and read my diaries about what my life felt like before, I can only say that this has been an inner trip for me. This has been living a whole different side of my nature and my life. It's just like being given a whole new side to my life, and it's always surprising to realize there were times when I felt either overworked or poor and that I didn't have any time to myself. When I look back, I think, "Isn't it strange that I could feel this way, and yet I know there were times when I was less happy?" One of the things that seems strange to me is how soon we forget our own experiences and how unaware we are of them at the time. It's as though once you go through a terrible grief, when it's over, you almost forget what it was like. I think that this is probably true with one's relationship with one's parents, when you read about some of the struggles in breaking away and growing up and how painful they were and how much hostility and antagonism one felt toward one's parents. Yet once this is gone, it's simply gone, and you completely forget the way you felt. I felt very unhappy with myself after Thomas was born because I didn't make more of the experience, that it wasn't more beautiful. I think that I wanted this third pregnancy so that I could perfect the experience, and it is very strange—it's basically the same thing.

Frank is the same, we live in the same area, and there hasn't been that much change in our lives. Yet in a way, it's as though I can reorder experience. It has nothing to do with the way things are, but the way one looks at them. That's part of it. Also, I have faced my own inner development, so I am quite different from who I was when Thomas was born. I have developed, in an inner way, a way that was previously undeveloped.

After Katherine was born, especially when Frank would say things to me like "Maybe you would like to get a job," I would feel bad and think, "Don't press me, don't push me. I want to do what seems like the right thing for me, and I'm not ready yet. I'm not finished with this experience yet. I haven't worked my way through it. I haven't found all the fulfillment." This time, I feel that I have. I wanted so much to have one baby wherein I felt happy. I think I feel that way now, and I think it took three children to do it.

I am struck at reading my diaries. First of all, I'm struck by the fact that as I started doing this in a systematic way, I began to see different connections among certain things. At first, I thought I probably would be able to do some writing before I have the baby and finish off things because I felt that after I had the baby, I wouldn't have any of the same feelings. I would be blank; I had to strike while the iron was hot. I don't feel so much that way now, and I feel that as long as I have this overall plan of what I'm doing, it doesn't matter whether it's done now or after the baby is born. I feel that after the baby is born, I'll feel just as much inner obligation to do this as before, and I find that keeping the diary on tape is a tremendous help. It's a safety valve, but also, it's a safety valve that doesn't take all of my time and energy. It used to be that in my life before, by the time I finished diary writing, there wasn't any time left to do anything else in the way of writing. There is always time to do something or go someplace or be involved in some other kind of distraction. I feel that I have plummeted to the depths of my own nature, and I feel that I do want to write a series on family, religion, knowledge, love, and creation. I saw this overall plan, this blueprint of what I wanted to do, in 1958 when I was in New York. I think returning to Boston was really a false creation. It threw me off as far as integrating my innate capacities, such as they are. But now, I feel this is a period of fantastic psychic integration. That's what I would call it. Now, I can go ahead with these five categories. I am amazed that I saw this plan because I had so many notebooks. I always had the feeling that I didn't know where to start. Now, I certainly feel that I do. I know now what I want to do. In reading the diaries in succession, covering year after year, from the late 1950s through the 1960s, I can see that my personality was a moon with a bright side and a dark side, and my personality turned from a full moon to the dark of the moon. I can see why the moon is my symbol; I have a feeling of something turning.

One of the things that used to bother me when I would meet somebody like Mrs. Bradshaw, who owned the Exit Shop, or Emily or Connie Stark, who does beautiful stained glass work, or probably even Winnie is that I used to think, "How can they do things that are so beautiful?" The things they make seem so beautiful and so happy. When I deal with material that is close to my heart, it seems ugly and destructive, especially if one is expecting the reaction of people who say things like, "Oh, I don't like to go to the movies unless they are lighthearted entertainment. Why waste your time on reality when there is enough reality around?" That always amused me. But I used to feel about myself, "Why do I write all this mournful, sad stuff when people like Connie Stark do stained glass that is so beautiful?" It seemed that whenever I wrote anything, everything was a nightmare. The anguish and the suffering after Thomas was born—this is a long wailing tale of woe. Yet I feel that what I want to do is something beautiful, and things can't be both beautiful and ugly at the same time.

It is strange to see my personality go from the dark parts to increase and increase and increase until they are the whole personality. They begin to spill out into every aspect of life and aren't confined to short periods of time, every now and then. In reading the diaries, I'm impressed, at certain times, with the care that I had taken to write things down and to outline things or put ideas down as though I knew that at some time, I would go over these things. It struck me that integration would be the key to the whole period. It seems to be a period of the most incredible integration—integrating the children, the house, my psyche, and everything.

For a long time after Thomas was born, I wondered whether I should have quit my job, and then after Katherine was born, I was in the hospital one day sitting out on the sun porch, and for some reason, I started thinking about whether I should have quit my job. I guess it's because that area around Columbia Hospital resembles Capitol Hill. I wondered if I should have given up my job. Then all of a sudden, like a flash, I told myself, as if

I heard a voice that said, "Well, maybe the Rotch Library. To give that up was different, but having once done that, the job at the Library of Congress didn't really matter." There was no point in trying to keep that job for any number of reasons. I thought it was interesting to feel that to keep the job at Rotch Library would have been different. It depended somewhat on the job, and the job at the Library of Congress was too surface an endeavor. I've had insights like that through this pregnancy. I've seen connections in everything.

It was a fantastic milestone to meet Mrs. Kotschnig. I keep thinking, at different times in my life, of the things I've wanted to do or study. I would like to read more things that Jung students have written and join a Jungian book discussion group, and I would like to write. I think that probably, I would be less interested in getting a PhD in library science. Frank has mentioned before that maybe, it would be a good idea if I did that and that it would increase my income, increase our joint income. But here's something else I keep thinking about. Having a baby is a rebirth for the mother. It's like high school again. I have a brand-new lease on life. I keep thinking about what I want to do with my life and how things seem different to me. I do think that children are a means to one's own self-development.

I don't think Thomas is going to the Montessori school. This is his last probationary week, and he only went one day this week. He wouldn't go this morning. It's difficult to know why. I feel that it probably has something to do with me. He feels that the baby is coming, or he feels that his position in the family is being undermined. I wonder if he feels rejection. Do I give Thomas enough time? Katherine Louise just demands time, and as Frank says, she begs to relate to me. She follows me around, and she's into things, and she's doing what I'm doing, whereas Thomas is much more inclined to go off by himself and do things like drawing. I think Thomas is absolutely a great boy. I wouldn't change him in any way at all. He's a fabulous kid. I've thought all along that he seemed very secure and never seemed threatened. I've always felt that he probably got enough, yet I do feel that if he had gotten more from me, maybe, he would be more willing to go to the Montessori school.

I think of my own kindergarten experiences of failure, and there are moments when I feel disappointed. I'm disappointed because it didn't affect me in any way at all. The only thing I remember is how disappointed my mother was, how my mother thought I would be illiterate.

Thomas really likes to go to Nona's playschool, so maybe, he needs to stay home more with me. I wonder if it's because I don't give him enough. Is time that I take to do other things time taken away from him? Is it possible to have any time to myself and still give him enough? Does he ever sense that I'm trying to hurry him into bed or that I'm trying to get him to take a nap so that I can get half an hour to myself? It's the only time that I have, and most of the time, either one child or the other child is up. Does he sense how crowded I feel sometimes? Does he feel that he's intruding on me or that I'm rejecting him? I wonder. Do I take enough time out to have fun with the children? I think that's very important. I know that Frank does. Do I? Is what I do for the children, just chores and drudgery, bathing and dressing them and cleaning up after them? Does it feel like that to them?

I returned two books to the library. One was the Bowlby book about the nature of the child's tie to its mother, *Attachment and Loss*. The other one was *Captive Wife* by Gavron. One of them stated that since the Industrial Revolution, there has been an effort to minimize the importance of mothering, almost to the point of pointing out that it could be done by a machine. Going hand in hand with that is the decrease in the amount of skin contact to denigrate the role of the mother. There is less and less skin contact between mother and child, and skin contact is important. One of them also said that life with children shouldn't be so different than life without children. I'd like to get Ashley Montagu's book on *Touching, the Significance of Human Skin*. I'd like to get that from the library.

A week ago, Sunday, the Bradshaws came to our house. Mr. Bradshaw is an architect, and he's going to draw up a five-stage plan for Frank. It's interesting to meet and talk to them. They're both very interesting.

This past Sunday, I tried to sew Thomas's white jacket because Minnie, the Real's dog, had bitten it in so many places. It was ripped, and I didn't have any white thread. I was so annoyed with myself because to have two children and not to have a spool of white thread seems unbelievable. Finally, I got some white thread, and then I started to sew on the machine. I couldn't remember how to thread the bobbin or whether to thread the needle from the back or the front. I had to get the instruction book out and was trying to do this while Katherine was sleeping. At the same time, Frank was fixing his Volkswagen signal light or the rear brake light, and he was so frustrated because there was something wrong, and he couldn't seem to fix it right. I don't know what the problem was. He was very frustrated. Then I got out the Sony cassette recorder, and I couldn't find the earpiece. I was frantically looking around for that, and all of a sudden, it seemed as though everything was out of my control. Everything was beyond what I could deal with or cope with or manage. I expected the whole thing to be broken. Everything seemed so hopeless or beyond me. There are often times like that, and it was raining, raining, raining, and raining. On top of that, Thomas was asking me if I would draw a boy and would I draw this and that. I felt as though I was ignoring him. I should have told him that as soon as I finished the sewing, I would read to him or draw. I feel that a lot of times, but I'm not sure that I always do it.

Mrs. Adams came this week and did a lot of things for me. In a way, I feel torn because it seems more hectic when she comes since I have to get ready for her. At the end of the day, when the house looks so much better, what a shot in the arm! It's fantastic. It feels so much better to look around and see some semblance of order.

I tried to get Carol Ann to come over and cut my hair, but I don't think that she's going to be able to do this. She's going to move from her apartment, and she doesn't know where she's going to be working. I'll probably lose touch with her. She's had so much hard luck.

I feel as though this time, when I go to the hospital, I'm going to call Emily, Mrs. Bradshaw, and Connie Stark. I'm looking forward to having a good time. I think that the little hypnosis that Frank has taught me will help me, although for the past couple of days, I haven't been able to get any finger anesthesia right. I feel that I can only deal with surface things. It's such a hurry to get this done and get this done and get this done that I can't go into anything very deeply. I can't take time out for hypnosis. It's like trying to run after a bus that you never quite catch, but I keep thinking that I'll just finish these few things that I have to do, and that will be all. I won't have anything else to do.

It's been the most absolutely marvelous pregnancy that anyone could possibly imagine. I've been so grateful to Frank for everything.

I was thinking about the children, and it's odd that sometimes, Thomas can be "tantrumy" toward me, not exactly kicking and spitting, but almost. Yet he can be with either Frank or his grandfather and he's the most civilized person. He acts older when he's with other people. I think the child's tie with his mother is such that his most primitive side is expressed to the mother, and to the mother only. It's very strange. I don't understand it, but I think that it does work that way.

Halloween, we went over to Frank's parents, and they had dinner for us, and the two children were just adorable. Katherine was a devil, and Thomas was a skeleton.

The day of our anniversary, we went downtown to a sale at the Store and bought a high chair and a lamp for the bedroom and a hat rack for Frank's office. The following Wednesday, we celebrated our anniversary. I called my mother on her birthday. Since then, I've had a letter from her. It's the strangest thing. I called her and talked to her, and she talked to Thomas. However, I had the feeling that I was keeping her from something, as though she was getting ready to go out or she had company, although I think that if she did, she probably would have said, "So-and-so is here" or "I'm getting ready to go out." I had the feeling that she was in a hurry to wrap up the call, and I have had that feeling with her for about five years, as though she's so busy with the surface things that she's doing and going to do that I can't really reach her. It's very strange. It may be a feeling that goes back to childhood, the feeling of not being able to hold her attention for a long enough time. But ever since I talked to her on the phone, she sent us a cute anniversary gift of four dishes with our names on them, and she has sent a letter. She does write to me more often than I write or call her. But she's very absent when I talk to her. It's like not reaching her. It's like going through the formality of calling your mother on her birthday or Mother's Day, a gesture without any content.

Anna called to wish us a happy anniversary. It was the same day that we went to Frank's parents, and it was lucky in a way. I had put Katherine in for her nap although she didn't sleep, so the result was that I was able to have a kind of long conversation with Anna. It was fabulous to talk to her. What was really amazing was that it was the first time that Anna talked so much about herself. I have always found it very stimulating to talk to her. Always, the conversation is punctuated by two or three books that I want to get and read. Anna said that her life seems to her a little bit like the swimming lessons that she took, where she learned all about how to swim and the whole theory of swimming but has never experienced swimming. I wish that I had asked her to elaborate more on that because I think swimming is a poor example—if that were completely true about her life, then she would be able to tell somebody how to look a book up in the catalog but wouldn't be able to do it herself. But there is something there, some quality that makes it possible for me to see why it does bother her. She talked about Jung, and that's what we mostly talked about, about how valid Jung seems to be. There is an analyst who's supposed to come to Boston after the first of the year. Most of the time, when we talked before, she had given me all kinds of food for thought, and this time, the conversation was different. Afterward, I kept trying to grasp what it was that she felt was bothering her, in her terms.

My relationship with Frank seems to fluctuate so much. Maybe, "fluctuate" isn't the right word. I can remember the time after Katherine was born, when she was about two months old—in fact, it was when Connie took that picture of Frank, Katherine Louise, and me—and I wonder if marrying Frank and having these two children was a mistake. Up until after she was born, I used to wonder that, but I don't anymore. I think that it was absolutely the best thing I have done. I suppose I could have married somebody besides Frank, but I think it was the best thing that I did marry Frank and have these two children. It's strange when I think of how after Katherine Louise was born, I wondered if I did the right thing, and now, I know that I did. Katherine Louise is the most beautiful thing that I've ever seen, the most exquisite experience in my life. It's probably the pregnancy, but there are times when Frank does things that hurt my feelings, and there were recently several incidents like that. Then on Wednesday, we went out and celebrated our anniversary, and it was the most amazingly incredible, truly and absolutely magical day.

November 15, 1971

I have so many things to say I don't know where to begin. Some of the things I want to say are left over from the last time I recorded. I was thinking this morning that the baby is due in nine weeks. It's strange. I keep thinking that this is the happiest time of my life. It's hard to imagine that I could be any happier. I find the feeling hard to explain. I feel that I'm beautiful. That's what it is! It is way more than happy, but I feel that I'm beautiful, and I feel that everything around me is beautiful. It's like seeing springtime although fall is my favorite season. I'm not as fond of spring as some people are, but it's as though everywhere, things are in blossom, the buds and the leaves. When I look at my dishes or rug or when I look out the window, the appearance of everything is enhanced. It's as though everything I see is also pregnant. Everything has a beauty, a glow, an enhancement, or an expectant air about it. I suppose I'm investing the most mundane things with something of myself.

When I think of how, after Thomas was born and, to a lesser extent, when Katherine was born, everywhere I looked, I could see the cracks, the peeling paint, the dust, and the cobwebs. Everywhere I looked, I saw evidence of decay, deterioration, and fragmentation. This is exactly the opposite, and the relationship of psychological and physiological is amazing. The changes that one goes through during pregnancy are so imperceptible that I hardly notice them. In fact, I can be tricked into thinking that I always feel this way. It's deceiving. I feel so great; it seems that's the way I always feel. Maybe, it has something to do with growth hormones or all kinds of things together.

Even the places around New Carrollton and Route 450, which I always find so depressing, I can drive through, and I feel insulated from everything. It is a very inner experience; my attention is always drawn inward and never goes out too far beyond myself. Probably, for that reason, things that don't touch me too much don't have quite as much effect. It's similar to the feeling of a beautiful day or an embrace. It's something wonderful in spite of the fact that I do find it harder to get around and harder to watch Katherine Louise outside. I also have spells of extreme tiredness. I'm probably more cross and more irritable, and there are times when I have been very hurt by things that Frank has either said or done. But when I do think about it at all, I realize how minor these things are and that even though I might be hurt at the moment, they do not hurt my basic self or my main stream of development.

The Sunday of our anniversary, we went downtown to the Store and bought a high chair and a bentwood rack for Bill's office and a lamp. It was a strange day. It seemed that whole day that Frank was mean to me. I had asked him about hypnosis, and he gave me a long lecture about my needing to be motivated, and if I didn't have sufficient motivation, I could never expect to make a success out of it. It was unpleasant. I had gone downstairs to do the laundry, and when I came upstairs, I fell, and afterward, I said to Frank, "I want you to know I didn't hurt myself," and he said, "Oh, nobody, nobody, kids. Everything you say has meaning." It seemed he didn't think that the house was clean enough. He was going to make pancakes, but before he was through, he banged around everything in the kitchen as though things weren't where he wanted them to be.

It's very odd. We went to Georgetown, and then we went walking in Canal Mart. It was as though I were some kind of adjunct. He picked out what he wanted, and that was it. I was going along for the ride, which means that I began to crawl into myself. That's not very good. As somebody said once, when you suppress hate, you also suppress love. It makes me feel gypped out of something. Every little thing was horrible. And yet you know we did do something together. When we got down to Georgetown, we walked along the Chesapeake and Ohio Canal, which is beautiful. We walked past the Doxiades city planning office there and went into the Canal Mart. We stopped in a bookstore and looked around there. It was a very beautiful day, but it was just not right. I could not seem to tip the balance in another direction.

The previous morning, which was a Saturday morning, we got up, and Frank immediately started to put pressure on me. Oh, he was late, he was late, he was late, he was late, and he didn't know whether he had time to eat anything. I got so flustered that when I cracked an egg for scrambled eggs, I dropped it down the disposal. The children were crying for attention. One was crying for one thing; one was crying for another. Then right in the middle of this, Frank asked if I knew where his hypnosis material was. He's totally disorganized. He never has any place for anything. He goes to a conference on hypnosis, and when he comes back with notes, folders, and brochures, he leaves them anyplace. I feel that I should put these things in file folders and file them away for him, but I don't have enough time. I only have time to watch the children. After he had worked me up into this state and made me rush and rush to get his breakfast, he sat over his coffee for forty-five minutes. My digestion had been so disturbed that I wasn't able to eat my own breakfast. Then he had an hour to sit down and relax. When he left, he said, "Well, don't be uptight. If you feel any tension today, why don't you go into a trance." I felt so angry that I'm even surprised at how angry I still feel. Furious, I feel absolutely furious, like hatred. I don't consider myself a tense person, an uptight person, a disapproving person, or a censorious person, but when he puts this kind of pressure on me and when he's so relaxed, I become one. When we are going someplace, while I'm trying to get ready, he's practically asleep, and we're late all the time for everything. And then, of course, he says, "Well, don't get uptight." That particular Saturday, I felt like a victim, an emotional victim. That was part of why Sunday was so bad. And I finally told him Sunday night how I was trying to get breakfast, watch the kids, and find his hypnosis material while he sat for a whole hour over a cup of coffee before he meandered off to work. When he left, I felt so tense. His image of me is so distorted that I felt like crying. I felt I had to wash the degradation off, as though I had poison on me. It was a horrible day, and it was our anniversary. I have two things that bother me in our relationship. One of them is that Frank treats me as though I am an authority figure. I told him about the guy that lives over on Joyceton Court whose wife left him. His girlfriend was over there the other morning, and they were moving stuff out. When I mentioned that, Frank said, "Well, he has a right to have a girlfriend. He has to sleep with somebody. His wife left him. So who's he going to sleep with?" I wasn't disapproving of the fact that the woman was there. I was telling him because I thought it was funny that the guy was driving his car on his lawn and that he seems to be such a surly person. Then I am put in the position of defending myself as if forced to say I don't disapprove of the fact that his girlfriend stays over there. So there's that. The other thing is that Frank seems to have a much lesser need to relate to people than I do. He sees people at work all day, but that's different. He's such a one-man band, all on his own, that I feel superfluous. He likes only the things that he picks out for the house. He would like to pick out the dishes and the glassware.

There's the incident about the draperies. I had asked him so many times if we could get draperies. We'll buy the draperies last, if we ever get them, because he'll pick out the things that he wants. That hurts me, and it makes me feel that anybody could fill my shoes. Like what am I doing here? I'm superfluous. I'm only the one that knows where to put things back when they get left around.

Maybe, it is a greater need on my part to relate to people, or it's that I don't really see as many people, and I'm not as deeply involved with as many people as he is. Deep down, I have a feeling that maybe, my taste is not as good as his. When I am looking at something, using my aesthetic judgment, and deciding if this napkin looks better with this or that placemat, I could probably be swayed and be convinced that my choice isn't the right one. I have doubts about my own aesthetic judgment, whereas Frank doesn't. He knows what he likes, and that's it—he doesn't care about anything else. It might take him twenty-five years to get what he likes, such as a turntable for the stereo equipment or bookshelves. Still, he wouldn't like it if somebody gave him these things. He'd turn up his nose, literally, at what someone else had given him. But he might never get around to getting the thing that he wanted himself. These are the two things that bother me. It's strange to see some of the things that bothered me so fantastically much in 1968, I mean, to the point where I felt paranoid. I felt that he was my enemy and that he wanted to destroy me, but now, I see these things more objectively. I'm still affected by them, but not totally as I previously was.

For such a long time, he has been saying that we should move the teak table into the kitchen and the round table into the dining room. Every time he makes a suggestion, it's always like "Why don't we put your father's bookcase in the basement?" or anything that is something that I had from before the time we were married. If it is something that someone has given me, he tries to get rid of it, or he covers it up so that he won't see it. Every time he walks by one of the chairs that go with the teak table, he bumps his toe and swears violently. These things feel like aggression that is directed toward me; he doesn't feel free enough to direct it right at me, so he directs it at these things of mine. I find it strange. I also find it annoying. He is so extremely haphazard himself about his own clutter and possessions everywhere. One object of mine and he'll immediately want to put it away someplace. He cleared a whole lot of my books off the bookshelves and made room for some of his own books. He just threw mine in a box in the closet, and one of the books he put in there was the dictionary, one of the books that is used fairly often. He didn't pick out any particular ones; he just made room for himself and his things. He keeps talking about how he's going to put the teak table in the library and how he's going to buy a table to replace it. It will be five years before he gets around to replacing the teak table. In the meantime, he doesn't even see it.

We went to Scan and bought a Rya rug. He did switch the tables and put the round table on the Rya rug in the dining area, and he's saying over and over, "Doesn't it look nice?" I think that he feels so frustrated in some areas in his work, such as dealing with his landlord at the office, that I decided that it doesn't really matter where the teak table is. It doesn't really matter if it's in the library or out here. I don't have a vested interest in its location. If it makes him feel freer and less thwarted to move all the furniture around the way that he likes it, that's okay with me because I'm sure that for years and years, I could have arranged the furniture any way that I wanted to arrange it. But why does he want to spend so much time on these things? Why doesn't he spend more time either at his office or on the office downstairs? But then that's his choice. It doesn't matter that much, but it would make me happier if he wanted to mend some of the things that we have. It is as though he'd like to be left alone. He doesn't want anybody to bother him. I wonder, in a way, why he wants a wife, and I wonder about his attitude toward my father's bookcase. My father made it, spent time on it, but that's probably being sentimental on my part. There's no reason Frank should like it or like it to be in the living room. I guess it just makes me feel two things: (1) it's a dead end to fight this out with him in any way, and (2) I should give my time and attention to the children and try to create something with them and with Frank, try to create something positive and good. Another feeling I have is that it makes me want to make the people that I have known, especially my father and my grandmother, live forever as though I'm going to take that little family, just my people, and recreate them so that they will never die. It's strange to want to do that. It's also interesting to me to see some of these things in relation to how I felt about them after Thomas was born. Maybe, I'm too sensitive to these things.

The Wednesday following our anniversary, we celebrated our anniversary by going downtown. Frank's parents stayed with the children, and we had lunch at the Port of Georgetown, a restaurant in the Canal Mart overlooking the Chesapeake and Ohio canal. The whole day was magic. It was absolutely magic. There were just the two of us in the restaurant. It was after the lunch hour, and to look out the window at the water and the leaves floating in it—it was a mild day—was fantastic. At that point, I had finished going over and sorting out all my notebooks, and I knew what I wanted to work on. I could see a number of things lined up that I wanted to work on. So many things have fallen into place.

When we left there, we found a shop called Exit, which had absolutely the greatest clothes that I have seen in a very long time. Frank bought me a brown tunic. It's a Moroccan man's shirt with embroidery on it around the sleeves and around the neck. The embroidery is in yellow, orange, and turquoise. We bought orange jersey pants to go with the chocolate brown tunic. And it was fun to meet Mrs. Bradshaw who owned the shop. Her husband is an architect, and he had designed the interior. It had built-in furniture, and the walls, the floor, and the ceiling were all the same color, kind of putty brown. I was getting a lot of attention. I felt like a spoiled child. Why should I feel so good just having attention lavished on me and getting some new clothes? It's strange. When Frank takes me out like that, he can be incredibly nice and also, at the same time, do things that hurt me so much.

We came home, and there was a big, big, big full moon. The whole day was absolutely tinged with magic. To look out that window in the Port of Georgetown and to look down at that drifting canal water. The canal is beautiful. I love to see it and walk by it and on those big old stones, like cobblestones, and see the autumn leaves on the sycamore trees and in the water. Autumn is my favorite time of year.

Claire, Frank's dental assistant, had also stopped over to see us. She brought her daughter Pam with her. It was interesting to see Pam because it's been a long time since we've seen her. They stopped in for lunch. It doesn't seem as though Pam is doing very much painting. I don't know why, but we gave Claire her wedding gift, a pewter bowl that we had gotten at Rockport. We talked for a while, and then they left. But whether it was because the moon was full or something else, I felt creative and happy.

Even though I am pregnant, at the time that I would normally have my period, there is a slight change in me. After having this incredibly creative period when I could see the work that I wanted to do and in what order, when I finally got out the few stories, the short stories that I did about a little girl, I read them over and looked at them very blankly. No ideas came. I felt tired. Nothing happened.

The Monday after the day that we went to the Store, that is the Monday after our real anniversary, I took the children to Zoe's for the day, and Zoe told me that she thought that they would not have any more children because the whole pregnancy with Andy was so full of recriminations that their relationship has never really recovered from it. It seemed quite sad to me because the one thing that Zoe's nature needs to flower is a home and children. Going over there, wondering if the car would start, having to manage the two children alone in the car, and taking care of the things that I had to do weren't easy, but it was a beautiful day. It had rained on Sunday night; it was misty, and then it got windy, and the leaves were coming down like snowflakes, so the ride over was pretty. Just getting out of the house and getting away from that Sunday situation, I realized something about the things that I have been fretting so much about with Frank, as though the two of us were locked in a telephone booth; if you work or do get out, it's as though the wind blows through your brain, and you don't see things in the same perspective. When you don't get away from your own situation very much, I don't know what it is, whether you begin to act out unconscious fantasy or whether you're much closer to your own unconscious because there is nothing else that intervenes. It was a breath of fresh air to get out, just the physical act of getting out and going for that long drive. It was such a nice day. Mrs. Adams had come. I felt different, especially after Zoe told me about her pregnancy with Andy, and I told her how happy I had been this time; I felt that Frank is good to me. These things that bother me, it's the proverbial tempest in a teapot or else it's like goings on in a pet shop, everything in a miniature world, except for the great big emotions that go around and around.

Last Saturday, November 13, Claire and Jim Roberts came for dinner. It was extremely pleasant and very nice to meet him. He is a lobbyist for Standard Oil in Washington. I asked him what his typical day was like. He said, "Lots of wining and dining."

In two weeks time, we're having Mandy, Frank, Hetty, Alfred, and possibly, Frank's parents the day after Thanksgiving. I was trying to find some *Gourmet* magazines, the November issues, which have great Thanksgiving Day recipes in them, but I couldn't find them. I began to be quite annoyed because Frank's closet is such an unbelievable mess. If there's a pile or anything around and I ask Frank if he will sort it out because they're his things, he'll take a paper bag and put all the stuff in the bag and then just stick it in the closet, like the books that he put in the living room closet. I can't understand why he'd put them there. He has no place for books, no place for slides, no place for his hypnosis material. This material just floats around everywhere and is always visible. All of a sudden, I started looking in the kitchen cabinets to see if I could find the issues of *Gourmet* magazine, and it turned out that there had been some book reviews from the *New York Times* in there, and they were not there anymore. I asked Frank if he knew what happened to them. He said, "Well, they might have gotten moved someplace. Weren't they in the bedroom?" I looked in the bedroom and suddenly became convinced that he had thrown them out. Of course, he wouldn't own up to it. He'd say, "Well, they might be out in the carport storeroom. Tomorrow, I'll look out there." I said, "Did you throw them out?" And he said, "Well, not consciously." He wouldn't consciously throw them out; that would be a mean thing to do. Was I accusing him of being mean? I said, "How could you throw them out and not know that you threw them out? How is it possible to do something like that and not be aware of it unless you had amnesia?" I was absolutely furious.

One night, when I was feeling sick and had gone to bed because I'd had a cold, sore throat, and cough for about a month, he came into the bedroom with my sandals in his hand and threw the sandals on the floor, as if he is the one who cleans up the kitchen. The thing that was making the kitchen such a mess was a pair of my sandals on the floor, but he leaves his shoes, sneakers, and socks everywhere. I trip over them all the time. Also, I had put decorations on a cake, and he took the frosting tips and threw them into the drawer and in a spot where they don't belong. I was sitting in the kitchen and saw him do this. It wasn't just that he did that, but whenever he does anything, even if he says he's going to cook breakfast, it's as though he's wreaking a kind of aggression on everything. These are either items that are mine or things that I have put somewhere; on the other hand, there could be mountain-high mounds of his clutter that I have begged him to move, sort out, or put away. But if it's his clutter, he doesn't see it. In fact, he likes to be surrounded by it. But if it's a thread belonging to me, he picks it up and throws it. That hurts me personally because it makes me feel unwelcome here. It makes me feel unwelcome in my own home as though I don't have a particular stake here or any influence. I was absolutely furious because I regarded that as similar to opening somebody else's mail. I began to get violently furious, and I decided that the thing to do would be to purchase the book review sections and send Frank the bill. Maybe, I'm being small about this or putting too much meaning in it. I don't know. I guess that in the end, it's not so much about the standards to which one holds other people or whether other people fall short or whether you are critical of something that somebody else does, but it's how much I can give and how much I can do in the present framework. Certainly, he does enough good things and provides enough, and I should be able to do a lot myself. Anyway, I decided that the thing to do would be to order the *New York Times*, and that would be that. I guess that's what I'll do and not fret about it anymore.

That whole thing about the *New York Times* articles is that I remember the night that it happened. It was the night that I went to bed sick. He wouldn't do it in front of my eyes because I would probably say, "You can't throw those away."

Without saying anything, in his body language, Frank acts as though he thinks that I don't keep the house clean enough. It's impossible to do anything more. What's strange is that the hours that I put in, as compared to the hours that he puts in, are far greater. The whole thing about the *New York Times*, and when I was trying to find those issues of *Gourmet* magazine, is that it's his family that's coming. The amount of time and the amount of effort that I will spend working so that we will have a nice time and then everything that he has is in such a mess that you can't find anything at all of his. It's a complete mess. All the closets are unbelievable. Anything that he has anything to do with is in shambles.

Down in the basement, you take your life in your hands when you walk down there. He still hasn't put the connection in to hook up the dryer. I have to hang all the clothes on a line myself and wait until they dry. Why doesn't he do some of those things? Why doesn't he finish off the basement? Why doesn't he connect the dryer? Why doesn't he get his other office going? Why is he so concerned about this very neat pile of articles from the *New York Times* that I have? Why doesn't he build a shelf for it instead of throwing it out?

When Claire is coming, he's ready to paint the whole house. There's no expense that he wouldn't go to or no effort that he wouldn't make—for instance, buying the Rya rug and moving the table over it. He was scrubbing the legs of the white chairs with an attitude that conveyed his opinion that the legs of the chairs should be scrubbed once a day. When I think of that night, when I think of the time when my sister and her little boy were down here, I remember Frank acting so awfully. He had a cold, but you'd think he was dying. When he took us to the airport, he was really horrible, absolutely nasty in the car. And the time before that, when my mother came down, he took her to the airport, but he was so late that she missed her plane. When my mother was here, he'd come home from work and immediately fall asleep on the sofa and not make the slightest conversational gesture. That's how he is about anything that I want to do or am interested in or anything that I want to buy for the house. If I want to get drapes, well, that can wait. Yet, if someone like Claire is coming, the amount of work that he does is unbelievable. What do you do under circumstances like that? I mean, how do I separate these feelings? I have to feel a certain way about myself. I cannot have Frank's view of me or what I think is his distorted view of me influence my sense of self. It can influence myself, but not influence my basic opinion of myself. I don't want to run Frank down, and I don't want to do things that will make it harder for him to fulfill himself or to do things. I don't want to curb him in any way, but it gives me, more and more, a feeling that I want to create beautiful things. It's the strangest thing.

When I look at those stories, those little girl stories that I wrote a long time ago, I want so much to create beautiful things. I also feel, when I do think about it, that the worst things about what Frank does to me is that they cripple my capacity to love and give because they make me feel hurt and make me feel squelched and unloved. In the end, it means that I give less.

When I think of some things, when I think of how I have treated myself, say, in the ten years before Frank and I were married, from age of, say, twenty-one to thirty-one, I ask myself, "Did I not do things to certain aspects of my own nature that were probably even worse?" I don't know whether it would seem like brutality to my inner nature, but the whole outer aspect of my life, the husband part of me, got top priority. Did I have the humility to face my own inner development? I had given myself to outer development rather than to inner development. I did that to myself. I can't blame Frank. These other things are minor, and I can't say that he does anything worse to me than I have done to myself. Why should I expect him to treat me better than I treat myself?

Thinking of the way that I felt after Thomas was born, I felt that Frank was trying to destroy me, trying to get rid of anything that was mine, annihilate me. I think that he is a person that has a minimal need to relate to other people. He is totally absorbed in processes. That's just him; probably, it's not that he's mean. So the impact of my whole personality on him would be some kind of intrusion. It is strange when two people are thrown together in marriage.

I've always had a lot of fears about myself; one of them is that I will be perceived as an authority figure. I don't want to seem fantastically disapproving of everything around me. I don't want to seem like that. Because I was the oldest in my family, I felt that my brothers felt that way about me, that I was always correcting everybody around me and saying, "Oh, look, you have dirty hands." So there's that, and then there's that other thing about aesthetic judgment. If I buy a dress, it wouldn't take much to have someone, whose aesthetic judgment I respect, tell me, "That was a mistake. That looks fantastically ugly on you." It wouldn't take much to throw me off, so to speak.

Last Wednesday was the day we bought the Rya rug for the dining room, and that was quite a nice day; Thomas and I had haircuts at Carol Ann's. I don't know whether it was because of riding in the Dodge, but whenever I get out of the Dodge, no matter how short a trip we have been on, I feel as though the baby is in a peculiar position, and I can hardly walk. Thursday morning, the veins in my legs were bothering me. It turned out that it wasn't serious, but I am sitting here trying to recover from the pain. Thursday morning was a strange, strange morning. It was horrible.

Tuesday, November 30, 1971

Today is Tuesday, so it was last Wednesday, the day before Thanksgiving, when we went downtown and got some bowls at the Store and bought a book on hypnosis and childbirth at Yes and came back. It was that day that I finally saw in outline form the way I wanted to do the short story I wrote called "The Room." I still wasn't exactly sure how I want to do it, but at least, I had an outline of all the things that I, at least, definitely want to include. Since last Wednesday, I have not had any time to work on it. Not only that, but Frank was home Thursday and Friday, and we had company on Friday. He came home early Saturday and was home on Sunday and was home a great deal yesterday. It's a real, real, real effort to get time to myself. We had Alfred, Hetty, Frank's parents, Mandy, Frank, and Robb here the day after Thanksgiving. And what is amazing is that I worked absolutely for days and days and days, planning the meal, making sure we had enough silverware, dishes, glassware, doing a few other things, and watching the children at the same time. I was very glad to see everyone, and some of the things I did needed to be done anyway. It still was amazing that the day they came, on Friday, I thought surely I would have had things planned well enough ahead so that I would have some time, but I didn't. We had a very nice visit from them, I think. Wednesday, we cooked the turkey, and then on Thursday, we cooked the ham. Frank changed the bedroom furniture around somewhat. The children had their baths, and then they did drawings at their little table, which is now out in the kitchen. Thomas and Katherine both did a drawing before they went to bed. It was Katherine's very first drawing, and she really did rather well. She kept at that one piece of paper for quite a long time. They were really cute with the crayons because first, one would monitor the other and say to the other one, "Here's one for you," and then a little while later say, "Here's one for you." In other words, the children weren't selecting their own colors; they were picking colors for each other and also giving the other the next crayon. Thursday, I felt tired, going from one chore to the next. We opened the UNESCO calendars that came and opened Frank's mother's birthday gift, the Waterford glass creamer and pitcher. We didn't open the birthday box in the end because it looked so pretty, but it was a day when I should have had a nap, but I never did, and I dragged myself from one chore to the next. We did call Foxboro and talked to my brother John and his family. They plan to stay in Foxboro. Thursday, I was feeling terribly teary and hurt. I guess it is a result of Wednesday night. When we came back from going downtown on Wednesday, going to Yes and the Store and to Saxatone where Frank bought a tape, we came back and went to a couple of supermarkets, and Frank stopped at the liquor store, and by the time, we got home, Katherine had slept just enough in the car so that she didn't take a nap, and she also wouldn't go to sleep until nine or nine-thirty at night even though she slept for what seemed like only twenty minutes in the car. The children seemed especially frantic. It was dark and rainy, and they were running in the house, and I was trying to do laundry and dishes. I felt exceedingly tired. Frank cooked the turkey Wednesday, and it was done at eleven at night. I cooked the vegetables. He helped me with everything.

Finally, the children were in bed, but not until ten at night on Wednesday. The turkey wasn't going to be done for a while. I had entertained the idea that I might be able to do some recording, and I kept thinking that maybe, I could take a nap, even if for just half an hour, and then get up and have the dinner. I had been toying with the idea of staying up late on some night to do some of my recording, but my hip was bothering me, and Frank kept saying that I should go into a trance. Finally, after Thomas went to bed, I felt cold. I felt as though I were coming down with a cold. I lay down on the sofa and just looked at the tree, listening to the rain outside, and thought, "This is what it means to be taken over by life. This is what it means to be completely used up by life." I was debating whether I should take a nap or go into a trance and take a nap and then get up. I decided, first of all, that I would try the trance, and no sooner had I gotten into a trance that the phone rang, and it was Frank's father. Frank talked to his father for a long while.

After that, Frank came back into the living room. He was reading a new paperback that he bought and said to me, "If you don't want the evening to be a washout, why don't you go into a trance?" I said that I was trying a trance when the phone rang. He said, "Well, just go back down into the trance." He was almost yelling at me, and finally, I started to cry. I felt so totally exhausted, and I felt as though he were just hitting me over the head with a tennis racket. I dissolved into tears. The tiredness got to me. Frank said, "Well, I'm not going to listen to that. You're just trying to make me feel guilty." He stormed out of the house and out the door and brought in some stuff from the car and then went downstairs.

When he came back, he got his book and sat at the dining room table. It seemed to me he was unnecessarily hard on me. I felt as though I hadn't done anything to him. I felt so tired, and it was so late. Midnight dinners aren't exactly the easiest thing for me being seven months pregnant; then he was punishing me by leaving the room and sitting out in the other room and reading his book. So I lay there feeling very sad that he could walk away and read his book as if his need for anybody else is minimal. It seems that he goes around in his own orbit. I felt bad because he had three days off from work. It's true that he had other things to do, but still, he did have a little time to use at his own discretion. It seemed that I had my regular duties plus more. All the other work we were doing was to entertain his family, which I am very happy to do. They have been very nice to me, and I'm very glad to do it. I couldn't help but think of the efforts that we have gone to when someone like Claire is coming or Frank's family and then what happens when my mother or my friend Connie comes. Usually, they miss their plane because he can't get up early enough to take them to the airport.

When my sister came with her son, Gary, Frank virtually dissolved. He got a cold, and he would come home and fall asleep on the sofa. I guess, I should realize that for some reason, he cannot make that kind of effort unless it's for something that he wants to do. He can knock himself out if Claire, his assistant, is coming for dinner, or his brother Alfred. He could tile the whole basement and panel it at the same time. If it's something you are expecting him to do or asked him to do or if it's about a relative of mine, then he falls apart and retreats.

I was thinking that I'm doing all these things and all this work and crying out of exhaustion, more than anything else, and being completely interrupted and frustrated at every turn, trying to go into a trance and have the phone ring, trying to get the children into bed and not have them go to sleep, this is frustration of your own will.

Eventually, the dinner was ready, and we did sit at the table to eat together. We wished each other a happy Thanksgiving and talked about losing weight through hypnosis. I was telling him about Lisa Griffin and what my sister had told me about her friend Lisa, her weight problem, and also how she had been brought up to suffer. After the meal, Frank was going to get us coffee. We sat in the living room, and he said he would get coffee in a minute, and then he continued reading. Thursday, I never recovered from the lateness of the meal and the tension between us, and that's why I felt so tired on Thursday. I went into the bathroom on Thursday to take a shower, and I cried in the shower. I thought it would be nice to call my mother in Foxboro, and I told Frank I'd like to call my mother, and he said, "Well, why don't you make a tape recording of the call, and then you tell them I said hi." I thought he wanted to listen to what we said, but then he wouldn't even say hello. I felt hurt that I was going through this effort to have his family here and he wouldn't even say hello to my mother. The other thing is the money. Frank worries about the long-distance call and how much it's going to cost and how long I'm going to talk. That seems to me so stupid. I thought he would say something like that, and I said to him that I would at least like him to say hello. Anyway, he did wish my mother, very briefly, a very happy Thanksgiving. That's why I cried in the shower because I thought that it is so unfair that I have to work so hard for the same thing and that he can work much less hard. The effort that we both go through to entertain somebody he wants to entertain or somebody in his family, but if I ask him to say hello to my mother on the phone, he acts as though he is put-upon. "It's going to cost so much. Why don't you write her a letter?" He likes to select his own social settings. For him, to make the slightest effort in a certain direction, when it's not something that he has initiated, seems impossible, and he doesn't seem to be able to do it. That made me feel very bad.

After my shower, I went on, but I was very tired. At least, I had everything done and thought Friday should be easy. It turned out that things weren't prepared as much as I expected them to be.

Thursday morning, I started to tell him that he makes me feel unwelcome here. If I can't cry in my own house, where else can I cry? It's such a drain when those things happen. Then he said, "Well, okay, we're not going to have any more people here. That's all there is to it. That's the end of entertaining," which is another one of his responses that annoys me because when I want to work something out with him, his attitude is "Well, if that's the way you feel about it, okay. We'll never go out again." It's one of these total solutions where he withdraws into a kind of ball. So I said, "Solitary confinement."

I did enjoy seeing everybody that came. I enjoyed seeing Robb and talking to him about the work that he does. He told me that he has started psychotherapy. To me, he seems such a sick person. He is very appealing and likable, but he seems so incredibly in need of help, and in a different sort of way, his sister, Mandy, does too. When I think of Hetty and Alfred and how they are both so intelligent and at the level of affluence that they have had all their lives, I can't figure out how they could have possibly done such a bad job with their children. To me, it's almost unbelievable.

Mandy is like an absolute copy of her mother. She refers to her mother as "Marmee" as though she were saying "Mommy" the way she did when she was three years old. She worships her mother, and I understand that her apartment looks just like her mother's. Robb seems incredibly ill. Alfred brought slides. I was impressed with his slides. They were terribly beautiful. It was hard for me to watch them because I was trying to watch the children and I was trying to get the dinner at the same time. But the ones I saw were beautiful, especially the landscapes and seascapes. He took some pictures of the Knights of Columbus building in New Haven, which, I think, was designed by Kevin Roach, and also the Frank Lloyd Wright building, the Marin County Courthouse in California. He has the eye of a poet. There's one picture that he took of his house; it was a side view that he took after a storm. He also took out some slides of the back of this house. They were beautiful, and yet I've never seen a photography book in their house, and I have never seen any of his slides enlarged and framed.

I had felt animosity toward Frank because he was so reluctant to say hello to my mother on the phone or to my brothers, and yet I can do unsparing and unstinting work to make the visits of his family pleasant. I did feel hostility; he doesn't really appreciate anything of me or of mine, and yet when I see Hetty and Alfred and I look at their children, I wonder if I could ever do that to Thomas. I wonder if I could ever make him like Robb.

Alfred's slides were exquisite. Hetty, who does paint as a hobby, can recognize beautiful things. She's never had any of Alfred's slides enlarged and framed for her house. Her house is completely devoid of anything that would reflect any of Alfred's interests, and the kids seem to have been given so little. Not only that, but Alfred has no books on photography. It's strange when you think of the things that people could do for each other when they're married and what it turns out that they actually do. Women can be destructive, cruel, and dominating. I don't want to be that way.

Somehow or other, on Saturday, I kept thinking about Alfred's slides and how nice some of them were. Some of the hills in California that were surrounded by mist looked Chinese. They looked like Chinese scroll paintings. It was interesting, the feeling of the Pacific that he captured. One has so much capacity for both creation and destruction, and I guess that's what it amounts to. I kept thinking about them on Saturday, and then Frank and I talked a lot about Alfred and his son, Robb. There is so much hostility between Alfred and Robb. They are interesting in a way. I don't think that I have read anything by John O'Hara, but I imagine that they seem like characters in a John O'Hara novel. They are so American, considering the small town in Pennsylvania that Mandy and Robb grew up in and the kind of parents that Alfred and Hetty are. But there is something about Hetty—I guess, it's her pathology—that seems so fascinating in a strange way, but she is somebody that could be written about. I thought, "My God, my God, my God, my God, I don't want to be like that, making everybody miserable and destroying everybody around me." Hetty is, well, you'd expect her to be like Andy Warhol's mother, or you'd expect Andy Warhol to have a mother like her. Frank and I did talk quite a bit about them and about the town the children grew up in.

Mandy had said to Katherine Louise earlier, "I'll give you a piece of candy if you give me a kiss." She said it a couple of times to Katherine Louise, and she said to Frank, "If you give me a kiss, I'll give you a piece of candy," and Hetty said, "Now, you know why I like to call you Candy." To me, it was just unbelievable because it was like bringing your daughter up to be a sacrifice, bringing your daughter up to be a piece of a chocolate bonbon, to be passive and consumed. It was so horrifying to hear that, but that is what it amounts to. I guess that's why Mandy seems so empty, so hard, so brusque, so bored, so utterly, utterly bored, so dead, so completely dead inside.

Frank and I talked, and I recovered somewhat from Wednesday night and the Thursday call to Foxboro.

Saturday, we went out and bought Thomas shoes. Sunday, Frank's parents came over for the afternoon. Frank's father brought the tape recording of the account he wrote of Katherine Louise's christening. It was nice to see them. We were at Zoe's last Saturday night.

I asked Myron, Zoe's husband, if he read Elicia Bay Laurel's *Living on the Earth*, and he dismissed the book with "Oh, it's really hard to live on a farm, and that book gives the wrong impression of life on a farm." I don't think it does because I don't think that's what it's trying to do. I don't think it's a how-to book on living on a farm exactly. It was probably his reaction that made me wish that Zoe could read that book because Zoe should write a book like that. Zoe does all these things so instinctively, like the plastic dishes that she has for the kids. She has a couple of dishes from Ursell's that are beautiful. The particular print that she has in her kitchen is an old-fashioned advertisement for Bensdorf Cocoa, but it looks as though it was painted by Aubrey Beardsley. It shows a woman in a kimono—it's turn-of-the-century art nouveau—and she has blond hair and is wearing a red kimono. The steam coming off the cocoa is curly, like all the lines in this print, but it's such a domestic scene. I know that Zoe has bought herself a book of Berthe Morisot's paintings, and Morisot has painted many domestic scenes like that. I've never known anybody that is so skilled in the way she picks out kids' books and the way she knows where there are great kids' toys. Just as Nancy Sirkus did on that book of photographs called *One Man's Family* about this woman, Frances Black, who has ten kids,

I think somebody could do a book on Zoe. Maybe, she's too instinctively that way. It's similar with Thomas asking me how you cut with scissors; it's a strange thing. I have to see the scissors so that I can see where I put my thumb and where I put my index finger. It's weird. I know how to cut with the scissors, and yet I'm not conscious of how I cut until I stop and make myself conscious of it. So likewise, maybe, Zoe is not that conscious of the things that she is doing. Somebody could do incredible photographs of Zoe and her kids. I began to think of a book called *Living as a Mother*. It would include things like the Berthe Morisot book, teaching Montessori in the home, it would mention Summerhill, creative playthings, the La Leche League, breast feeding, and some of the books that I think are whimsical, something like that issue of the magazine that Anna sent me called *Equals One: The Child Equals One*, something that would mention good books to read and some of the material that would help you get pleasure out of motherhood. That was one idea that I had.

Monday was a strange day. It rained all day, and Frank felt that his day was a total washout. He went to work in the afternoon, about three. He did go to work in the morning, but then he was home for lunch for a long time. It was as though he started working at three in the afternoon, and then he went to the bank and did the shopping. I let Thomas stay up probably too late. Last night, I was going to do some Christmas cards. I wanted to start writing them. Because Frank was here most of the time, Katherine didn't take her nap. She did go to bed early. By the time I did get to sit down by myself, it was very late. I don't feel quite as tired as I did last week, which is wonderful. I hadn't done any more on my story, "The Room," but I did address some of the UNESCO calendars that will be mailed out as gifts, and I did do a few cards last night.

Today, Frank went to work at about 1:15 p.m. I put Katherine in for a nap, and Thomas went into the room and let down the side of her crib, so that got her up, and he brought her out here, and he said, "We want to make a house." I put them both back in for their naps, and they went to sleep, which was convenient. I feel that there's another person in me that's waiting to be let out. It's strange—a shadow that's ready to come to the fore. Maybe, that's similar to what Frank said when he used to feel that he was like Janus, two-faced. I feel that, except in my case, one is much more of a shadow figure than the other—they are not two equal figures.

Because we had the picnic table up here for our guests on Friday, it was still here on Sunday, and Frank's mother suggested we use that in the kitchen. Frank has mentioned that to me a couple of times. Why don't we just try it in the kitchen? It's really the strangest thing. He wanted to put the teak table in the library, and he said that then we could take the lamp from the living room and put that in the library. I wondered whether I am paranoid. It seems to me as though the few things that I have here, that I had before we were married like the bookcase that my father made, the little table that my father made, or the bookends that my father made, Frank is always suggesting to me that we put these in the closet as though they're intruding on him, and the same is true for the teak table. In a way, that teak table has been the bane of his existence. I don't want to feel that I have a vested interest in the table, that it can't be moved from one spot to another. I do think it would look like nothing here in the dining room. The round table looks nice because it recapitulates the roundness of the hanging lantern, which hangs down from the center, and also because there is a round rug under it, which makes a big difference. It gives a focus to the area. The teak table looked nice in the kitchen, especially with the light shining on it. It looked great. I had this strange feeling that Frank wants to take the teak table, the lamp that I used to have on Charles Street, my father's bookcase, two filing cabinets, the bureau that I used to have, the red desk that I had selected and put them all in one room, and then he could tie a rope around the room. I think it's weird. In my weakest moments, I have fought against it. It used to make me nervous when he said something about the table. He hates the chairs that go with the table. My father's bookcase, that's what I feel worst about. That's the possession that I prize the most because my father made it, and it's something to hold books. I feel bad when he says, "Why don't we put that in a closet?" Every time he brought these things up, I used to feel strange as though he were pulling the rug out from under my feet, and usually, he would say to me then after that, almost in the same breath, "Why don't you get a job? I could watch the kids Tuesday and Thursday mornings. Why don't you get a job?" I feel that he was trying to destroy me. These things always come up at the same time. He wouldn't mind being at home. He wouldn't mind doing what I'm doing. I used to wonder why that bothered me because I do want to work as a librarian, especially when I think of the life of a housewife. I do have interests, but there's a difference between feeling that you want to do something yourself and feeling that you're a victim, and I feel on guard about that, almost as if I'm going to find myself doing things that I don't really want to do if I'm not very careful. I want to make sure that they're things that I want to do. I don't want to be a tool.

I do feel about myself that I have never been used, that I'm almost unuseable because I don't make myself available for that, and also, I do feel that I have done more or less what I wanted to do. I don't feel the way Connie felt, as she has told me before, the feeling of having absolutely no control over her life. I do feel I have control over my life, and I feel that I am the architect of my own life. If I've never done anything or developed my own potential throughout my life, I can't blame other people. It would be my own doing. I also feel that I have, to some extent, brutalized my own nature. I have let one side take precedence over the other side, and I have done that to myself. I seem to be very wary of anybody else making me a tool, using me as a tool or a victim. But I have done this to myself, and maybe, I've done worse things to myself than anybody else has.

Nevertheless, it gives me a peculiar feeling when Frank starts talking as though he were going to make a heap of all these few items that I have, like the prints that I have, like Winnie's drawing of me that I like very much, Winnie's prints, and some of the other possessions I have.

Frank has lost weight, and he's so happy about it, and he should be because of his age. He's getting into the heart attack age, and it's dangerous to be overweight and do the kind of work that he does. He feels great about it. He has discovered a newfound control, and he seems now to be much more the way he was when we were first married. He has much more energy although he says it's probably because my energy is decreasing that it seems he has more.

Because of the things that have ensued about these pieces of furniture, I think that he must have felt upset the day the moving van pulled up to his apartment and dumped all my stuff there, including my clothes, and the way he so resisted moving from that little bachelor apartment into the other apartment at Cherry Hill. It's strange when you think of it because all these things are symbols or reflections of some inner world, the melding of his things and my things. I felt, when we were married, that he would have preferred it if I appeared naked and possessionless, just a blank. That's why he can make me feel unwelcome or as though he doesn't value anything of mine. I think to myself that I could make something destructive out of this. On the other hand, I have to value certain things myself if there is something that I like. It's up to me to keep it or have it where I want it. Everything just points to the fact that I have to exert myself more. I decided that probably, it's a great thing to have the teak table in the library. I would like to get a Rya rug for the library, keep the filing cabinet in there, and set it up as a study. Maybe, that's the only way that I will ever be able to get any recording done because one of the strange things about living both here and in Cherry Hill is that any place where I lived with my family, I could always go to the kitchen. I could close the kitchen door and make coffee or sit down at the table, and that way, I could at least be up when the rest of the family is sleeping. Anywhere that Frank and I have lived, there wasn't any way that I could get up in the middle of the night without disturbing Frank. There is no way I can turn on a light here in the living room or in the kitchen without having the light shine into the kids' room. Maybe, this means that there will be a little place to go to if I do happen to have a few minutes and everybody else is asleep. Maybe, it is great to have that room in there with the portable tape recorder. Previously, I would have to record in the living room, and I always felt so self-conscious when Frank was there although I don't mind him listening to what I record. I always want him to look at it when at least it's typed. Maybe, I should get a Rya rug for the room. Probably, we should get the children's furniture first. Maybe, that will be worthwhile. Maybe, I can turn this into something positive. At first, it would seem peculiar to me to have a little room that is a replica of my apartment on Charles Street, but that's the thing, I think, that is also so weird about most of the houses that I see where people live. People who live in houses have so little that reflects any interest or any activity—no darkrooms, music rooms, or greenhouse rooms. There's just a room for eating, or two rooms for eating, there are many rooms for sleeping, and then there is the room for the television, and that's it. Maybe, it would be great to have a little room that I can go into and get away. I would like to get a good lamp for that table. Maybe, it will be a great thing. I can use it at night or, maybe, when Pam, the babysitter, is here or when the new baby comes. I will be able to go in there. I won't have to sit in the living room at night, where there are no drapes, and feel terribly exposed to the street.

Friday, December 3, 1971

Time is going and going. Today, it looks so much like snow. It looks so wintry. I think snow was predicted. The children are outside with Pam. Thomas just came in for a cracker. I've been writing Christmas cards. I still have a few more to do.

Wednesday, we went to Dr. Kuhn's. We had an extremely pleasant visit. Frank came into the office with me. When we were coming back from Dr. Kuhn's, Frank didn't feel very well. It sounds as though he's coming down with a cold, and he's in such a bad mood that I wonder whether he is worried about something else or that other things must have happened. The past couple of nights, he has gone to bed early because he didn't feel well, and I've been writing Christmas cards. I have always enjoyed sending Christmas cards to some people, the people that I like to think about, certain friends that I had at different times in my life. When I send them Christmas cards, it's a little visit with them, especially if I have a letter or card of theirs to answer. I think about what I want to say, and it's quite pleasant.

This year, for the first time, it has seemed that the same thing doesn't quite turn me on in the same way. It's not exactly that the writing of the cards is purely mechanical, because it isn't that. It's not a mechanical operation, but I've felt so complete in myself that the things these different people represent or what I project onto them I no longer need because I feel complete inside myself. Yesterday, we had a call from the Montessori school, and they said that they had an opening for Thomas, that, in fact, he could start next week. Somehow or other, that gave me a strange feeling because I realize that once Thomas starts school, the kind of singular influence of the parent is over, but more than a feeling that I don't have the same

143

influence over him is the feeling that the major influence that I'm going to have on him I've already had. There is no going back. He'll be four in March, and if I had to do it over again, would I do it any differently, and would I be a better mother? I wonder if I have given him enough. That is the main thing because he's definitely at a point where he thinks about things; he feels things, and I realize that he has already taken from me the major things of his life.

When I think about my mother and me and the things that influenced me so much when I was younger than Thomas, I wonder, "Have I been happy enough? Have I given him enough of the feeling that he really enhances our lives, that life is fun and a joy?" It was strange to get that call.

Also, as the time gets nearer for the baby to be born, it gets harder for me to get around and also to get around with the children, all the winter gear that they have to wear, getting myself dressed and bundled up, and then going outside in the cold, just walking or standing around. It's a lot harder now, so we spend more time indoors. It's so strange to be with two children that age all day long, especially on days when they don't take naps; because their activity seems so random, they're so noisy, and the pitch of their voices is so high. After a while, I am looking forward to the time when they will go to bed and sleep. They are constantly pulling things off and out and then dropping them. They are into everything. I feel that I can almost do nothing except watch them. The reason motherhood is so hard in a middle-class setting is that there is no privacy for the mother. There is no privacy.

Monday, January 3, 1972

It's surprising to me that it's been a whole month since last I have recorded. There have been so many things that have happened and that we've done I don't know where to begin. I feel that time is running so short, that the baby is going to be born so soon, and that there's a terrible rush to do everything that I want to do before the baby is born. I don't remember feeling this way so much before Katherine was born, but I do remember feeling that way when Thomas was born because I was working on a bibliography and couldn't stop working on it. I feel the same way; only this time, I'm going over some of my old notes and diaries.

This whole pregnancy has been the most amazing experience for me. I see connections that I had never seen before. I see the connections between things and the relationships more easily, and maybe, I feel closer to my subconscious.

I was surprised that one morning, after I woke up, I was thinking about the fact that in 1958, when I finished my master's thesis at Columbia University, I had just finished reading *The Education of Henry Adams* and the idea came to me to write *The Education of Katherine Murphy*, about a girl growing up. I saw the book organized into five concentric circles: family, religion, knowledge, love, and creation. Between going home to Lonsdale Street, then moving to Charles Street, and then going to England for a year, I made many beginnings. And every time I was involved with a man, it altered the whole picture. Each time I was emotionally stirred, I would have different ideas about things. The result was that I had an enormous pile of not even beginnings, just ideas and maybe a note here and there. I had a few notebooks, but I hadn't thought much about them. Then one morning, I realized all of a sudden that I wanted to get out those five categories and that I wanted to do something in each one. I could see the way a little more clearly. Not only that, but I saw some individual stories, like the story about the pencil, a first instance of self-awareness, and the story about the room, having something to do with relating to one's environment. Instead of those ideas being scattered here and there, they were lined up clearly before me, like stepping stones.

I decided that I should organize my notes and do an inventory, and then I'd be able to work on these one at a time. I worked on the short stories that I had started before. Then, all of a sudden, it occurred to me that the reason that this outline didn't come and carry me along in 1958 was that I expected, when I went back to my parents' home on Lonsdale Street, that somehow or other, I was going to be able to affirm and participate and make up to my family for the fact that I had gone to Simmons College, that I was going to be the prodigal daughter returned, but that did not happen. Instead, my return was a complete failure. The result was I moved to an apartment on Charles Street. Therefore, I realized I couldn't think of returning to Lonsdale Street in 1958 as a kind of creation. I didn't see, at the time, that it was not a creative experience. It was a false creation, and it was a false start. Then it took me a long time before I got back on the right track again. It was probably not until I had children. I found it amazing to think that in 1958, my going back to Lonsdale Street was false creation. This then made it possible to think in terms of a whole lot of other stories that I had started as fitting into more of a total picture of pieces that I would like to do about a girl growing up.

In addition, reading through my notes led me to see this as false creation. I thought of the difference between my life in the ninth grade and my life in the tenth grade; I think I could have died in the ninth grade. That was the year that my mother had a stillborn baby. She went to the hospital on my ninth-grade graduation day. Earlier that year, I had had a strep throat for three months, and my mother was sure I had TB. It was a dismal year whereas the tenth grade was absolutely the opposite. I had friends, like Peggy O'Higgins, Millie Morrissey, and Marjorie Marshall. I got a job at the Massachusetts General Hospital. I got good grades, and I had stories and poetry published in the *Item*, the school literary magazine. It was amazing. I started at the job in the tenth grade. I'd go to Boston by myself, and I had something of a life on my own. I started my diary for the first time, and that summer, I had been to New York. I spent a month in New York with Jay, my aunt by marriage, and I think that was one of the milestones of my life. She did so much for me. It's strange too because my mother was so mad that I stayed there a month. My mother felt betrayed, felt that I really didn't appreciate her and what she had done for me, to think that I could go off like that.

When I saw the difference between those two years, I could see that it had something to do with the parental image and the fact that in order to grow up, you have to break away from home. I felt so guilty and felt that I was a monster for wanting to go to college. I felt so terribly guilty about this that it took me years to recover from it. I suffered for what should have been looked upon as something quite normal. I can see why it must have been so hard for my sister, Louise, to try to break out into some kind of independence. When I look back, I had such enormous feelings of guilt that were truly incapacitating for such a long time. I also saw how happy I felt having been to New York with Jay and then starting high school and having friends and being able to go here and there and having a job, besides babysitting jobs.

Naturally, one follows the path to happiness. I used to wonder how it was that I had outer development rather than inner development, why my whole inner life was so associated with my mother, and why it was always so depressing and incapacitating. I could see the difference between the ninth grade and the tenth grade, why I followed one bend, how what I thought was going to be creation turned into false creation, and how the result of that was that I went even further in my one-sided direction. Going to England for a year was going as far as I could go in one direction. It could be called ego development. It was necessary, finally, to go back and recoup my forces or remarshal my troops, and then the suffering was very painful. I made enormous strides, and in some ways, it probably never would have happened unless it was forced on me in the same sense as having Thomas and going through what I went through at the Cherry Hill Apartments, the utter desolation and agony that I went through there. I emerged from that a completely different person. Maybe not a completely different person, but I feel that I have synthesized so many inner and outer abilities. I feel I have woven almost all of my capacities into one. That has been one of the amazing things that happened to me during this whole period of going through my notes. There's always a temptation to stop. Maybe, I should work on this, or maybe, I should go on and read and read and read. Many things are associated with the mother-daughter story, where you can't plan, and also the story "Death," and the backgrounds for some of these stories are in some of my diaries.

I decided that the best thing to do would be to continue to go through the diaries. Then any thoughts that I had, I could get down and put into some form. In a way, it's like getting ideas for two more things. When I have written about how I felt at other times in my life, it strikes me that we're so unaware of our own experiences. It seems terribly self-centered, as though one could become completely trapped by one's own feelings, impressions, and emotions. I'm sure that this is true. On the other hand, it does seem amazing that you can go through a period of wanting something, like wanting to go to college, and then when you get there, you feel that's not what you want anymore. You really can't remember that there was something at work within yourself, propelling you into this situation.

I think the same thing is true with marriage and children—the urge that is so strong yet so many people, I should say women when they get married, don't remember—how much they thought they wanted this at one time. I think that it's even truer for other kinds of experiences. We're only partially aware of our immediate experience at the particular moment—like Ernest Hemingway's description of drinking red wine, then having the hot sun beat on your back, then going to a bull fight—and then there's almost no memory for the experience. That's amazing to me. I find it so revealing.

I'm up to 1961 in rereading my diaries; I guess I should consider the diaries to be on the same level as knitting. At any rate, it's fascinating to me that there are connections and insights into things that I see. I feel that after the baby is born, all of this will go. I'm so intent on doing this that I don't even want to stop to record it. I have very little time.

It seems that Katherine Louise, if she takes a nap in the afternoon, is up late at night, and Thomas is no longer taking naps in the afternoon at all, so the chances of getting a whole hour to sit down by myself are quite slight, and I don't see any other way. I feel that when the baby is born, all this will be lost, so I feel that I want to make the most of it now. It's a feeling of things opening up all of a sudden. It's like looking up and having a whole new view even though you are in the same spot or like being able to see around a corner. It's been a fantastic inner trip.

The birth of the baby is scheduled for January 17. I wouldn't say I want to continue the pregnancy any longer, but I certainly do want to make the most of this time because this will be my last pregnancy. It has been the nicest one of all, the most beautiful, and it's been such an utterly fantastic experience. I feel that I love everything. I feel as though I love the house, the view from my windows, and the Rya rug under the dining table, and I feel so incredibly happy, absolutely, incredibly happy. I don't know how I am going to cope, but I do feel very happy. I feel happier than ever before in my whole life.

Connie called me the other night, and I asked her if she had read the 125 pages of the motherhood tapes, and she said she found them almost unreadable, that she thought the editing job was overwhelming, more overwhelming than writing would be, and she wondered why I didn't get some kind of Dictaphone machine. I said that there was nothing on this subject, and she said, "Oh, there are millions of women. I saw an article in a magazine about a woman journalist who was in her thirties and who was married to a man who had been married before, and she had a baby and was really surprised that the baby would have to be delivered cesarean section; she told of her experiences being checked into the hospital and so on." Connie said that there were many things, but she couldn't think of any titles or authors right at the moment. She said that she knew that there were many on the subject, and that if I thought that I had written something about what was important and universal about motherhood, I hadn't done that. She said that if I wanted to do that, what I'd have to do is research. I was quite interested in having her comments, but they reminded me of so many times when I have shown Connie things before. She always says things like, "Well, that's good therapy, but it doesn't have form; it's not fiction," Anyway, I was quite happy to have Connie's comments.

There have been so many nice things that happened. Toni sent me an absolutely beautiful letter, which came the day before Christmas. Christmas for me is an utterly magical time. I adore Christmas. It is an inner experience, and to be pregnant during this season is a double inner experience. It's like having everything flowingly beautiful; it's more than I can stand. Everything is pregnant, swathed in life.

Toni sent me a beautiful letter, which came the day before Christmas. In addition to that, a few days after Christmas, she sent me a little booklet of her poems. It's a beautiful job as far as printing is concerned, and there are collages. The poems are in French, and the title of the collection is *Last Words*, and I suppose they're last words about Quechee, Vermont, but I haven't completely deciphered all of them. I was moved to read her poetry. Another thing is that I called Mrs. Kotschnig and made an appointment. Frank and the children and I went over there last Wednesday. I went in and talked to her while Frank and the children waited outside in the car. I feel that meeting her is one of the milestones in my life. I asked her about becoming a Jungian analyst, and she said she thought I probably could if I wanted to. She didn't think that my experience was all wrong for it. She is the first Jungian analyst that I have met, and to me, it was truly amazing. She gave me the book *Aspects of Love*, and then she gave me two issues of the magazine called *Inward Light*. She is an older woman, and it was for me an unbelievable experience to meet her. It was a real opening and something that added to my general happiness. Christmas this year seemed very subdued and inner. Last year, our cards all had messages of economic deprivation, how people were out of work and losing jobs and one thing or another like that. This year, although I think that the economic situation is probably either the same or worse, there weren't any of those kinds of messages, but we got fewer cards, and the messages all seemed low-key and inner as though they were more spiritual in some ways.

We got a beautiful card from Emily a couple of days after Christmas with music by John Cage. I finally realized that she probably made the cards she has sent that are like that—the one that was her wedding announcement, the Vietnamese artifact card that she sent for Christmas a couple of years back, and the Indian hand card with the sign of the Indian greeting on it. Zoe sent a beautiful card, John Birchfield's *Orion in Winter*, which I just love. Anna sent a beautiful card, and she said that she has a fantasy to do a collection of readings on the spiritual meaning of women or human liberation. It's such a joy at Christmastime to hear from friends. We had people the day after Christmas, including Frank's parents, his brother, the Goodmans, the Listers, and the Reals. I talked to Anna on the phone, and she recommended some books to me: Barbara Hanna's *Striving Toward Wholeness*, Anelia Jaffe's *Myth of Meaning*, and James Hillman's *In Search*, which has a final chapter on inner femininity. She mentioned Eric Neuman and how he feels that we need a new ethic based on wholeness rather than one based on the idea of goodness and perfection and that the new ethic is for man not to want to be any worse than he is but also not to want to be any better than he is. Anna mentioned one time, when we were talking, that she thought I was too young at that time to know that one is capable of evil, and I didn't ask her whether she thought I was old enough now to know that I am capable of evil. She said that there was some value to darkness and evil and that the dark side of oneself is to be redeemed and lived with, and she mentioned that Christianity is the task of every person to deal with goodness and that when she was in India, she could feel that this is true. In the West, this has been assimilated, and therefore, one can go into something else. She also mentioned that Jung said civilization hangs by a thread and that thread is man's psyche. She said that there's a Jungian analyst coming to Boston after the first of the year and that she's going to see this person then. She feels that she has a monkey riding on her back and that she doesn't really experience things, that she understands but doesn't experience them.

For Christmas, Frank and I gave his parents a print of Childe Hassam's *Boston Common at Twilight*, a reproduction from the Museum of Fine Arts in Boston, and for her birthday, we gave Frank's mother an Irish Waterford crystal creamer and sugar bowl. We had a very nice day. Frank's parents came over and had lunch. For Christmas, Frank's parents, in addition to giving us the TV set, gave me some Gwen Frostic cards, which I like very much. So all in all, it's been the most beautiful Christmas so far. For the New Year, I haven't made one single resolution. Maybe, it's because I'm too happy. I don't know, but I'm simply not making any.

There are moments when I feel so tired, and there are moments when I feel I'm going crazy, when the children are just unbelievably into everything and I am trying to keep up with them, to keep up with the next thing they are doing. Not counting those moments, I feel unbelievably happy. The pregnancy gives me happiness.

Ellen Roberts called and is going to come to see us, probably sometime in April on her way back to England. Thomas, although he has been home from school for a week, seems to like the Montessori school. Zoe and Myron came over the day after Christmas, and Zoe brought me a Kathe Kollwitz's book of reproductions. She brought Leo Lionni's *Alexander and the Wind-up Mouse* for Thomas. Most of her innate capacities are integrated into being a mother. The Sunday before Christmas, Frank and I went to Lesley Branck's for an open house, and I saw Myron and Zoe there, and another woman from the library. The event was quite nice. Lesley had a little boy that died last February, which was very, very sad. Today, I expected Mrs. Adams, but she didn't come. I always have mixed feelings about that because I have the feeling that I will have a few minutes to myself, like today when I've done this recording, which I don't have when she is here. But on the other hand, it's a different kind of boost when the house gets cleaned, especially now when it's so close to the time the baby is expected. It is hard to do everything and get ready for the baby. I should feel quite lucky that I have time to do any recording at all. Frank has been, mostly through hypnosis, dieting. He has lost quite a bit of weight. He seems extremely grouchy. I don't know whether it's because of the dieting, but Frank acts as though I'm not really doing enough for him or I'm doing something wrong or something isn't right; otherwise, it wouldn't be that way. I've tried so many different things to no avail. But I'm so happy that Thomas seems to like the Montessori school. I hope it continues.

Monday, January 10, 1972

As things now stand, the cesarean section will be performed at 9:00 a.m. next Monday. It seems odd to have it so calculated and scheduled. It wasn't like that with either of the two children.

Time is running out. I don't know why exactly, but I feel it's a rush to get certain things done, although almost everything is done, I guess. I had hoped that Mrs. Adams would come, and I had hoped that Carol Ann, my haircutter, would come. The upshot is that rather than having so many things to do myself, there are arrangements to be made with other people. As far as Carol Ann and Mrs. Adams and the babysitters go, there's not much point in trying to make these connections beforehand. I'd rather have a little time to myself. Time is running out. Things are really hectic, and I do want to have a little quiet time to myself before I go to the hospital.

Yesterday, I went to see Dr. Kuhn, and he asked me if I would like to have a tubal ligation done when the baby is born. After I left his office, Frank and I were talking about it, and Frank raised the question of whether this was irreversible. Does it have any effect on bodily processes? Today, I called Dr. Kuhn, and he told me that sometimes, in about 20-25 percent of the cases, there is irregular bleeding and that sometimes, maybe because of this, there are ovarian cysts that form. I called him back again and asked him whether further surgery was usually necessary. He said, "Well, probably not," but I wonder. I keep vacillating about what I want to do. I had thought that it might be a good idea to have it done until it looked to me as though it could probably lead straight to a hysterectomy, with the cysts and irregular bleeding. It is weighing on my mind. I have until

Thursday morning to decide. Rosemary, the nurse, is going to send me the form, which has to be notarized, in the mail.

Thomas has refused to go to Montessori school, and I feel guilty about this. I talked to Mrs. Ziachetta today, and I'd talked to Mrs. Harold before, and I'm going to talk to her again tomorrow. Mrs. Ziachetta said, "Well, maybe this is a difficult time for Thomas because he senses that the new baby is coming, and he may be under a certain strain." He doesn't want to go. Instead, he wants to go to Nona's playschool, and he wants to go to Nona's every day he said. He says various things like he doesn't like the children, he doesn't like Ms. Liberman, he doesn't want to go, and he wants to go to Nona's because Gregory goes to Nona's.

I have to get Thomas ready for school in the morning as though he were a package or object—feed him and dress him and rush him out. Most of the time, it's even more hectic at noontime when he's getting ready to go to Nona's because by that time, Katherine Louise is crying and fussing, and Frank is rushing around getting ready to go to his office. I am trying to get things done, yet I have an inner urge to sit and mull over my experience because it seems this is the last chance I'm going to have to even think. Maybe, it seems as though I have rejected Thomas, or it seems as though I've withdrawn myself from him. He definitely seems not to want to go, but when he comes home from the Montessori school, he seems to be able to do the most fantastic things to antagonize everybody. He's really aggressive toward Katherine Louise, and he acts out at the table when we have lunch. It's very strange. He acts like a different kid. He acts as though his ego was fragmented. Either he acts like the bully boy or he regresses to being like Katherine Louise and starts talking baby talk as though his ego is too fragile to take the load of all this and all these new things and to know who he is in the midst of all these things. When he's away from the Montessori school, he seems to be his old self.

His drawings have become very figurative. He's drawing people now, and they are beautiful drawings. He'll ask me if he can do a drawing. Saturday, he did one of the most fantastic drawings of Santa Claus. Yesterday, he drew some figures of a family, and they were quite amazing. His play is very involved, and he has a fantastic imagination.

I got him a little book about Benny the Giraffe, and he was talking about Pennie and Benny, so I let him do some recordings of stories, and it's amazing the way he'll sit down and record them. He was so delighted to do it. When he finished, he said, "That's the end of my talk."

The two children are so different. Katherine Louise is so different from Thomas that it's almost unbelievable. Thomas is not that interested in anything involving the environment or, in general, the domestic environment. He plays with toys much more than she does and watches television, certain programs that he's interested in, like *Sesame Street.* Katherine Louise, on the other hand, does all kinds of things that are her versions of what I do. She takes silverware out of the silverware trays and puts them in the dishwasher and then takes them out of the dishwasher and puts them back in the drawers. She loves to play with the dry mop, loves to do dishes at the sink, or comb her hair. Her toilette is very involved. She loves to run into the bathroom and go potty, although most of the time she doesn't do anything. She likes to have her hair combed. She loves to brush her teeth, loves to eat the toothpaste, loves to wash her hands, and loves to change her clothes.

In the morning, she gets up and wants breakfast, and right after breakfast, she comes out with an armload of clothes and tells me, "My clothes." She's very possessive (my clothes, my chair), and she names all the things in the environment and classifies them (Daddy's sock, Daddy's shirt), and when I'm going through the laundry, she's naming all the things that belong to different people in the family and who owns what. She's become very attached to her dolls, and she'll take Raggedy Ann, whom she calls Raggy Ann, to the window to wave goodbye to Frank. She'll sit Raggy Ann in the chair, she puts her in for naps, and if she doesn't, if she hasn't had her dolls for a little while, she'll start looking for them. She's very much the little mother. She looks after Thomas and does things for him. She knows where almost everything is in the house and can find just about anything with ease. She's very interested in the body and bodily processes and things like combing her hair and brushing her teeth and washing her hands. She'll take down her doll's pants and get Vaseline and Desitin to put on their bottoms.

Thursday, January 13, 1972

It's difficult to believe that in a few days, I'll be in the hospital with a new baby. This has been the most absolutely fabulous pregnancy. Even at the end, I feel that it could go on forever, and every now and then, I become afraid that maybe there will be something wrong with the baby. Then I think, "Well, no matter how hard it is afterward, I will always be thankful the baby is fine, and that is my only wish now." I have felt so well, and oddly enough, I feel as though I have more energy than I do in my usual state. I feel younger somehow; it could be because of the baby being a new person or growth hormones or something else.

Everything I look at gives me pleasure. I look out our front door at the trees across the street, and they all look beautiful, or I look at the duck decoy next to the green lamp, an antique duck decoy, that Frank got for Katherine Louise, and that looks so pretty. If I remember correctly, after Thomas was born, after the birth of the baby, I only see the dirty smudges, the marks, the fingerprints, the cracks, the holes, the rips, and the tears. Beforehand, what I see is everything knitted together, new connections all the time, or new possibilities. It's been truly the most amazing experience. Being pregnant is a fantastically selfish thing. It's a feeling of being all to oneself, like having a private world or a beautiful secret or a hidden garden somewhere where you can go.

There is the feeling all the time of wanting to clean out all of the cupboards, clean out all of the bureau drawers, sort out everything, as though I were going to die. That has prompted me to start reading through my diaries, and this has allowed me to sense the amazing connections of things. I saw the way some of the early things related to some of the later

155

things. Whenever I tried to do anything previously, I was always bothered by the fact that I didn't see things clearly in novel form, in play form, or short story form. It was the form that defeated me. With the advent of Women's Movement, I learned that all these forms are male forms. The form doesn't matter to me now. I'm going to do what I have to do and in the way that I think is right for the material.

I've had so many liberating experiences. The first one is that I can have anything typed that I want to have typed. This opens fantastic possibilities. I know what I want to do and can see an order to what I want to do. Each thing will have to be taken in its turn. I'll certainly spend a certain amount of time on the form, but I don't feel hemmed in by those old categories anymore, and this has been a fantastic liberation. I feel tremendously excited. I do, that's all.

The past few weeks, I haven't stopped. Any time I had the chance, I got things in order and, now, have made an outline of what I want to do. There are about six things that I can see clearly that I would like to work on. I don't know whether it was because yesterday, there was the full moon, but now that I have finished all the arranging and organizing and I have my six things, I have come to a dead stop, so I decided that today, I would record.

The past three weeks have been quite eventful in other ways. I had to take some antibiotics because I had a terrible throat. I don't know what it was, but the last time that I went to Dr. Kuhn, he gave me a prescription, and my throat seems to be a lot better, though I still have nasal congestion. Physically, I am finding it harder to get around, and sometimes, I feel incredibly tired. It's unbelievable. To produce three children in such a short time, it's difficult to imagine the amount of energy that it takes. When you think that most women have their children in their twenties, it's as though the cream of their energy is scooped right off, and it's probably not noticed because these women are so young, but a fantastic amount of energy goes into making a baby.

Sometimes at night, when I'm trying to get the children to bed and they are resisting me and Katherine's crying and Thomas doesn't want to go to bed, I ask myself, "Why would I want to have a third child?" I can hardly manage as it is. When I am with Zoe, I can see that she does have a lot more energy than I do, and she can be constantly on the go for longer periods than I can. Sometimes, I remind myself of a salmon. It's a strong instinct that propels me along to have another baby. I want to have this baby because of the experience of the pregnancy. The physiological and psychological changes are so fantastic that I wanted to have a pregnancy one more time, and I wanted to have it perfect. Still, there are moments when I feel as though I am like a salmon, that I'm going to make it through the delivery and then just die of complete exhaustion. It's as though the drive is going to kill me. The whole thing seems so fantastic. I also have that feeling that I am riding on the crest of a wave, and it's all going to go crashing.

I thought after Katherine was born that I would hit rock bottom, the way I did after Thomas, but I never did, not for as long nor quite as low. I remind myself of a spawning salmon. I find doing the work that I have to do and caring for the children takes everything, except the little bit that I give to this recording.

We had Myron and Zoe over one night, and Frank bought crabs. It was quite pleasant. We talked for a long time. Then, last Monday, I took Thomas and Katherine over to Zoe's. We spent a day together, and it was a beautiful day. I feel so proud of my two children. First of all, I don't feel that I am their equal. I feel they are so much better than I am. I don't feel equal to them, and I feel so proud of everything about them—their looks, their intelligence, their happiness, and just their total beings. I feel so proud that they are my children, so immensely proud of them.

It was interesting to go to Zoe's. I met her father and her stepmother. Zoe's apartment is fabulous. Myron is working very hard on his drawing, and Zoe said she thought that probably, they would not have any more children because the pregnancy with Andy was so unpleasant and that they have not overcome the recriminations over the conception and pregnancy. She does such a truly splendid job. I think she does a much better job than I do. I could say that I don't know why that's true, but I think there are probably a lot of reasons: she has books for the kids, and she's got their toys completely organized. I could imagine somebody making a movie about Zoe as a mother. I think the woman who wrote a book on Frances Black, the black woman who has ten kids, lives in New York, and is on welfare, could make a film about Zoe. What is so incredibly strange to me is that she has been hurt in the area that is her best area, as far as her pregnancy with Andy being horrible. Zoe fully comes forth in the area of being a mother and having a home, and that's where her wings have really been clipped. The irony is cruel.

Sunday, January 16, 1972

It's so strange to think of what will happen tomorrow. I feel so great now. I must give Thomas more.

January 17, 1972

On January 17, Monday, at 9:00 a.m., the baby was born cesarean section, delivered by Dr. Kuhn, and the baby is a girl. We decided to name her Jennifer.

Wednesday, January 19, 1972

The baby is an exquisite girl, perfect and beautiful. Above all, I wanted a healthy, normal baby, but I did have a slight preference for a girl. I told myself, "Never mind how hard it is; as long as the baby is healthy, be grateful." I have never been so happy. I don't want to lose the euphoria of pregnancy, the feeling of completeness, wholeness, everything being integrated and knitted together. I love Frank even more than ever. I feel that only now am I beginning to appreciate him. The children have given me so much. It's as though I didn't know it was okay to be happy. More than that, I didn't know that you are supposed to be happy.

Thursday, January 20, 1972

Excruciating headache up until 1:00 p.m. today. Mrs. Ripton and Mrs. Jacknicki, the nurses, came in to see me about it. They had wide-open faces. There was a program last night on channel 26 on learning disabilities in children—coordination, perception, and behavior. There was another on the San Quentin gas chamber. I must do so much more for Katherine Louise and Thomas, so much more love and stimulation.

Friday, January 21, 1972

Frank came today, and we talked about Dr. Kuhn. Frank said that Dr. Kuhn won't look him in the eye. Frank brought me *Living the Good Life* by Helen and Scott Nearing. Having the baby is like having a core drop out of my psyche and soul. It makes me feel like an anxious doughnut, like a ring of worries around an empty center. I read a very interesting article on aging from *Coming of Age* by Simone de Beauvoir in *Harper's*. Zoe called me, and today, I received a beautiful Kate Greenaway card from her. One spot on my varicose vein hurts, and my incision is beginning to hurt. The baby would not feed tonight at nine. I couldn't get her to wake up. I think we'll call her Jennifer. I keep worrying about the vein, the incision, breast feeding, how I'm going to manage at home, how I'll ever find Carol Ann. I saw the *Blue Angel* on TV tonight. It was superb. I reluctantly leave the waking state.

Sunday, January 23, 1972

I feel so beleaguered by irrational fears. I feel worried and anxious about everything. I wonder if there is any chance that the baby could be a mongoloid. Emily says she almost looks oriental, like a Cambodian dancing doll. I still have my headache. Now, it is in the front of my head. My breasts are tight and tender, and the beginning of each nursing hurts. My incision is sore; in several spots, there's draining. The outer vaginal area burns when I wash it. My left leg hurts. I feel so apprehensive. Tomorrow, the stitches come out. Otherwise, everything is fine. I've come a long way. I fight going to sleep because I feel as though I woke up from a bad dream, so apprehensive, so anxious. I worry about Thomas and Katherine Louise, especially Katherine Louise because when I call, she's either crying or Frank is scolding her. I feel like an elevator shaft that has lost its elevator. The core really has dropped out. Uncle Mike and Dot called today, also my friend Anna.

Wednesday, January 26, 1972

I had a very pleasant visit with Emily yesterday. We talked about the Women's Movement. She says there is terrific hostility toward it. She mentioned meeting people at bank parties and how these people start telling her all kinds of things. I think she finds this a very big drain. The last time I saw her, she said much the same thing about her students. She seems to be suffering from too many intense relationships to which she gives too much. Emily appears so fragile and so understanding that I can see how people impose their emotional state on her. I have done the same thing myself, and it's as though she doesn't have sufficiently developed ego boundaries. The way she lived with Pierre, when I first met her, she needed someone to hide behind. There is no central core that has an existence or momentum of its own there. She keeps getting sucked into other people's lives and keeps shunning other people. I guess that's why I feel I can only go so far with Emily. I guess that's why she is always disciplining herself and apportioning her time just to keep herself from the people who have desks near her at the Library of Congress.

Monday, February 7, 1972

That was all that I wrote while I was in the hospital. The last bit I wrote while I was waiting for Frank to come and pick us up and take us home. There were many things that I jotted down about the experience, but one of the most amazing things to see was the reaction of Katherine Louise and Thomas to Jennifer.

We came home on January 26, which was a Wednesday. Both Thomas and Katherine looked kind of unbelieving, and Katherine held my hand. I was in the wheelchair. Her eyes opened so wide, so unbelievably wide, and she held my hand and walked along beside me. Then coming home in the car, she leaned over the seat and kept trying to touch the baby. Thomas was interested but from more of a distance. Very soon after we were home, Katherine kept playing the little trick where you put your thumb between your fingers and pretend you have somebody's nose. Katherine kept saying that she had the baby's nose, and then she was very interested that the baby had a nose and that the baby had eyes, hands, fingers, hair, and a face.

The children never left my side while I was holding the baby, and they're still doing that. They say to me, "Get her, get her." They tell me when she cries, and they don't want me to put her back in her cradle to sleep. It's very strange. This whole experience has been much easier than the other times.

I recognize so many of the feelings I have now as similar to those I had before but now to a much lesser extent. One of those feelings is fear and an increased capacity to imagine harm. These are feelings I manage to keep in check most of the time. With the first child, the feeling was much more out of control. I feel myself being squeezed into a smaller spot. It's a fear of everything out of doors and as though there's something lurking in the outer darkness. Everything seems frightening. Every little while, I panic. I imagine that Jennifer has a cold. I imagine that things are going to happen to the children. I imagine that Thomas is too much in his own world. There is the underlying fear, the feeling of being very, very close to a bad and frightening dream.

The baby is three weeks old today, and I have so little energy. I am beginning to get cabin fever here in the house. It is therefore time to do this recording. This is the first one I have done since I've been home. I hope that it's not too much. It seems very hard to do. The first time that I start to write or read or send cards to people, it's so hard and seems to take so much energy and time. I hadn't expected to feel so weak.

My stay at Columbia Hospital was uneventful, except for the unbearable headache I had for several days because the anesthesiologist tried to give me an epidural and some spinal fluid leaked out. As a result, I had a fantastic headache; I also had some trouble with the vein in my left leg. I thought the Columbia Hospital for Women seemed better than the other two times, less like an institution. It has a more personal atmosphere, and the nurses there are incredibly compassionate.

Ms. Thompson, the nurse, was still there, and we talked about her sister who is head of the District of Columbia welfare agency, and another nurse, Ms. Louder, who grew up in Georgetown and took care of me when I came back from the operating room. She seems so Catholic. She had been to Catholic schools. For some reason, I had the feeling that her personality wasn't integrated. Mrs. McKensy was the LPN who took care of me on a minute-by-minute basis, and she was fabulous, and then Mrs. Jacknicki was the nursery nurse. The nurses all had immense praise for Jennifer.

One day, Mrs. Jacknicki and Mrs. Ripton came in to see me about the headache that I was having. It was so peculiar to be in bed and behold these two people looking at me; they had such wide open faces. They were perfect nurses. They were efficient, but they had such empathy that I was struck by the sense of the hospital not seeming to be an institution. I guess it's because of the kind of women working there and the general atmosphere. It was strange and wonderful.

I had far fewer drugs this time. I don't know what I was getting before, but I was high on drugs; I had highs on the drugs, and of course, afterward, there was a big letdown. This time, I had fewer powerful drugs, and I stopped taking them sooner.

I talked to Shirley on the phone, and she told me how she lost her baby in the eighth month. It is difficult to imagine such a loss. I talked to Claire, who told me about her operation, the hysterectomy that she'd had. My friend Emily came in to see me about three times, and I suddenly realized, when Emily was talking, why she feels she cannot come out here to see us. The people who have desks all around her at the Library of Congress can use up a lot of her time, so she forces herself not to talk to them; otherwise, all her time would be taken up by them. People at the bank too, and the parties that bank people have that she goes to with Pierre, exhaust her, and sometimes, she feels devastated afterward. Well, it suddenly struck me that she doesn't feel that she has the time or energy to come out here and see us. It takes a whole day, and that's too much. I also thought about what she had said about her first husband gradually cutting people off; it was strange because I could see how she could do that or how she could at least want to do that. I think that explains why I have always felt that I can only go so far, that there is a certain barrier there. I was thinking that the only way that you could not feel that way would be if you had something going of your own, which has such drive and momentum and was absorbing enough, that you felt you could provide counterbalance of your own to the demands of others.

I wrote to my friend Toni. She had sent a letter that arrived the day the baby was born saying she had a feeling that the baby was born. Anna called. She told me that Ann Bedford Ulanoff's book was out, and she told me about the new Jungian analyst that has come to Boston.

It's so peculiar to feel the place where the baby was; it's a big empty space. I'm so much more aware of it now than I was the other two times because my recovery has been faster. I'm back to normal much faster than I was the other two times, so now, I can compare it better. I want the secret place where the baby was to always be there and not go away completely. I think that's all I'll record of this for now.

Tuesday, February 29, 1972

We just got back from taking Jennifer to Dr. Molning's office for her first checkup. She is six weeks old, and Dr. Molning said she seemed absolutely fine and basically very healthy. He seemed to think that perhaps, she hadn't gained as much weight as she might, and he suggested that I give her four ounces of Enfamil every day. We came back, and she went to sleep. She's sleeping now, and I put Katherine Louise in for a nap. Thomas is out playing with Gregory, and Frank has gone to work, so I thought I would catch up with my recording. I've been keeping notes. I didn't think it would be as long as it has been before recording, but Katherine Louise is not taking a nap very much now, and I decided that if I were going to do any recording at all, I was going to have to plan it so that at least, once or twice a week, she took a nap. When she does take a nap, she's up very late, but last night, she fell asleep about 5:00 p.m. and woke up about 7:00 p.m. and was up very, very late. It doesn't really matter that much. There is not much point in keeping her up based on the theory that she'll go to bed early and sleep all night because that doesn't always work.

I have a lot of things that I want to say. It has been six weeks and one day since the baby was born. I remember the last time I recorded, which was February 7, and that was three weeks ago. I was amazed that after I recorded for ten minutes, I felt exhausted. I had decided to record because I had a lot on my mind. I had notes. I want to get these thoughts recorded, but after a short time, even my voice was tired. It's a little bit frightening to me to feel that I am overextending myself at a time like that when perhaps I shouldn't, but I feel so much more energy now than I did then.

One of the things that has struck me when I first came back home and the first several days is that Frank did everything as far as getting up in the morning and watching Thomas and Katherine Louise and getting breakfast, but as I began to do more, I found that I would come out to the kitchen in the morning, and I would feel tremendous hostility, absolute fury. Katherine Louise and Thomas had dripped honey all over the kitchen, or they had tried to make toast, and there was a loaf of bread broken up into little pieces all over the kitchen, or there was a glass of milk spilled all over the floor. Everything in the kitchen was sticky, and all the dishes from the day before were here and there. To walk out in the morning into this mess made me absolutely furious. I was filled with a fantastic fury. I felt like a mad woman, as though I were going to start beating everything into place, picking up the dishes, throwing them into the sink, getting sponges, and scrubbing off all the surfaces. I began to think that maybe, hostility is an aid to recovery because when I was getting back on my feet, it's as though I cannot stand the way something looks, so I get up and do whatever needs to be done even though I feel that I should probably be resting. I should be taking a nap. I should be off my feet. I should be in bed, but I see this mess, and it's just more than I can stand, so I tackle it with fury, this vengeful fury. If none of this bothered me, I could sit back and rest, but there is something that forces me beyond what I can do, but not too far beyond what I can do.

There were times I felt that I was overextending myself, and then I would cut back. I would feel that at least, I have done all of the dirty dishes, so maybe, I had better get off my feet now. It's interesting, this kind of balance between activity and doing things and pulling back and not doing things, but I was amazed how much hostility I felt. I also felt fury at Frank for leaving shoes, socks, and clothes everywhere. When I have made a gigantic effort to clear off one little space, Frank would come in, and five minutes after he'd been here, it would seem that a cyclone went through the place. That seemed to be the case. I was surprised at this feeling of hate or hostility in myself, and I thought maybe, it is an aid to recovery. I was also struck by the fact that I felt this in the morning, usually when I got up. I didn't feel it all the time, mostly in the morning.

There were many, many very pleasant experiences. On the whole, I feel that I have lived out my urge to have children. I felt it a little bit after Katherine was born and after we moved in here and a couple of times when Frank said to me, "Why don't you get a job?" It gave me the strangest feeling. My reply was "No, I'm not ready. I haven't finished doing something yet. Don't rush me." Besides, the feeling of living out this urge was there; there is also the feeling of wanting the experience to be perfect to the extent that any life situation can be perfect. I felt that I was so unhappy after Thomas was born, and I wouldn't say I was unhappy after Katherine was born. I wasn't, but there was still something left over from the experience when Thomas was born.

I always remember the Thanksgiving when Connie came here in 1969. She took the photo of baby Katherine, Frank, and me when the baby was two months old. I remember well thinking to myself that day, "I wonder if I did the right thing in getting married and having these children?" I was still asking myself that. I wasn't really that sure. But this whole pregnancy, I was absolutely sure it was what I wanted, and it has been a very happy experience, really beautiful. I can't see how it could have been any more beautiful as far as the relationship is concerned. It might be nicer if Frank had a million dollars, but I don't see how the pregnancy could be nicer, and so I think to myself, "Why is it the other two experiences or births weren't like this one? The children were equally healthy. The father was the same person. How could it be that one of them was such a miserable experience, that the second one was sort of nice, and the third one was just so fantastic?" It was delivered in the same hospital, and the first two were very close together in time. I didn't feel that things about me were any different inwardly. During the third one, it was as though I had arranged my experience. I arranged it so that I would have a certain experience. It was like arranging things in my mind, arranging my mind like an instrument, in such a way that unpleasant things or frightening things are glossed over, similar to the saying, "Keep your eye on the doughnut and not on the hole." There are certain peaks of joy, and I stay on one peak looking forward to the next peak, and then all the things that happen in between, I leap over as much as possible. I don't dwell on these things. I tell myself they are just transitory.

It is peculiar how the same experience, that is the birth, could be so pleasant, rewarding, fulfilling, joyful, and great the third time when the other two times weren't so. The operation, the doctor, the pain were the same, but it's as though I told myself beforehand what I'm going to feel, what I'm going to experience, and that's what I did. I don't quite understand this in myself. I don't like to think that we preordain things or that we work things out beforehand so that everything works out just the way we plan it. If so, we'd never have anything like a new experience. Nevertheless, I felt that I did arrange to have a certain kind of experience, or I arranged in my mind so that I'd experience the birth in a certain way. I feel that I can do anything that I want to do. I feel immensely free, and I think it's because I feel so inwardly free. I felt isolated by Thomas's birth and, to a much lesser extent, by Katherine Louise's birth. I felt I was no longer as free as I used to be, and now, I feel that I am much freer than I ever was because I am inwardly free, and I feel that I can do anything that I want to do, absolutely anything. If anything, the children have given me more strength to feel free, and this has been especially so with Jennifer's birth. I'm just so grateful that she's healthy and beautiful, and she's just absolutely perfect. I don't know how I would feel if she were ill, but I do feel that I can do anything that it is in me to do.

On this matter of arranging one's experience, part of it is a question of control, and the third birth, motherhood for the third time, was an experience where I felt I had much more control over the situation so that I could arrange my experience; I had enough control so that the frightening parts were less frightening. I never felt out of control, and that's why I recovered so much faster. One day, when Dr. Kuhn came into my hospital room to see me, he said, "Well, you seem to have things pretty well under control."

I think there is a tendency in me to want to repeat the experience until I master it, and that's why I always used to wonder whether I liked school because I made such an effort to master the experience that was originally so utterly, utterly, utterly frightening to me. I do think that my experiences are very much like what they used to describe in World War II, when men would have nightmares of living the battle scene over again. The men go through them in their nightmares over and over again in an attempt to gain control or mastery over a situation in which they had no control, and so it seemed to me the only way to gain any control was to repeat the experience until it was one in which I didn't feel very much out of control, not for long. Maybe, that's why it was a much better experience. Maybe, it's just a matter of control.

I also feel so much more love for Frank. There are times when I do feel hostility when he leaves stuff everywhere. Those are momentary things, but it seems that I love him so much more. I can see the enormous effort that he has made and, on his terms, how good he is to me and how wonderful he is to the children, but mainly, I see the enormous effort that he has made. I can see him doing things and trying to do things, and I think that I appreciate him more than I did before. But that makes it so much nicer—to feel more love for Frank.

This has really been a very pleasant postpartum period. After Thomas was born, I read in the book *Expectant Motherhood* by Eastman that the postpartum period should be a pleasant one. It should be as pleasant as the pregnancy. To me, it was a nightmare. I thought, "How can he say this? How can this man in this book say that the postpartum period should be a very pleasant period, as pleasant as any other period in your life?" But this time, it has been a very pleasant postpartum period, and I've lived long enough to experience what I thought was impossible to experience, even though I was surprised that it took several days to write, read, make any effort, and concentrate. In the hospital, you think in between feedings; you'll have a couple of hours. Isn't that great? You can write announcements or write notes. I had notebooks with me to read, and I also had a couple of notes to write, and there were phone calls I wanted to make. I forgot how, after something like that operation, it takes an enormous amount of energy to concentrate, to even think of making a phone call or making the effort to do something simple like get your handbag, get out your address book, look up so-and-so's number, arrange your bedside stand so the phone is right there, and dial the number. After the phone conversation, you feel completely exhausted. The first two times I tried to write, my handwriting looked awful. I was writing announcements, and I thought that they looked terrible. Reading or even following something on TV, it's really surprising how much effort is involved in trying to follow something in sequence so that even though I had little periods of time to myself, I was surprised that most of the time, I could only vacantly vegetate.

The day that the baby was born, I was taken out of my room on a stretcher, and there was a woman across the hall from me who was going home that day. She came out to say goodbye to me. It was peculiar because she was smiling at me, and I felt that she wanted so badly to relate—she was begging to relate to me, and I couldn't even smile. I was on my way downstairs for the operation. I didn't want to talk to anybody, other than Frank. I certainly didn't want to have a chatty conversation. She was looking at me, and she had a rather beautiful smile. She had said that she had had four cesarean sections, and the nurse said, "Four cesarean sections!" I said, "Which one was the easiest?" She looked as though what she had undergone was really something traumatic. It was too bad in a way that I couldn't have talked to her more because at any other time, I would have enjoyed talking to her, but at that time, it was almost weird that she was standing there looking at me.

From the window of my room, there was a row, a city block of old nineteenth-century three-story brick houses, and at one end of the block was a tiny V-shaped park with two or three benches. There were three or four derelicts sitting there. This was January—it was very cold—and the derelicts, who were men, were sitting huddled together. I suppose, if it were warm in the summertime, they would have been, each one, on a single bench. I thought, "I wonder what it's like to be out sitting on a bench like that, and at night too." I suppose, at night, they can get inside some doorway. Isn't it strange that they're huddled together like in a zoo where you see one animal on top of another? They're trying to feel the warmth of another human body, to be less lonely. Isn't it amazing the difference between the kind of lives that these derelicts lead and the life of somebody like Dr. Kuhn, who is so fantastically active and productive and does so much? These men are able to do nothing at all but sit on benches. It seems to me that it would be so hard in the wintertime to sit out on a bench and to be homeless. That's the worst punishment that one could possibly be given. It seems no job or marriage could be so horrible that life sitting out like that on a bench would be preferable to it. Maybe, it's just that I don't like the cold.

It was really strange to talk to Thomas and Katherine Louise on the phone when I was in the hospital because I'd very seldom talked to them on the phone before. Thomas asked me if I would still be his mommy. Then he told me he had sesame seeds and was going to plant them in the backyard. I watched a TV program about a woman who runs a nursery school. I don't know exactly what she does, but she is very impressive. Several other people were with her on the program, and they sang and danced. I think she wrote the songs, but I'm not sure. She's an immensely attractive person. She really looks like one of the new women. I think also that Juliet Mitchell, the friend of Cooper, the man who wrote the *Death of the Family* was there too, and there were some other interesting people. Gloria Steinem is quite amazing too. I saw Odets's *Paradise Lost* and *The Life of Lorraine Hansberry* on TV.

One night, when I was suffering from the unbelievable headache that I had because of the failure of the epidural they tried to give me, I watched a program on children's learning, and it showed kids that had a lack of coordination or who had something wrong with their perception or their behavior, four-year-old kids who couldn't skip. I began to think about Thomas and wondered if he had any kind of problems. After that, there was a program on the death penalty. It showed the death row cells at San Quentin. These two programs, to me, were scary, but a lot of the time in the hospital, especially when it got dark, was frightening. There were times when I felt my bed was a little boat in the ocean, and I was squeezed into one spot, huddled into one spot, as if all around me was a menacing ocean or a menacing darkness and as though there was just one little spot of day or one little spot of light with a fantastic ocean of darkness and I was just one little spark. Everything seemed scary; it was like waking up from a nightmare and finding out you are really in your own bedroom, and you're so glad you can turn on the light and see all these safe and familiar things.

One of the programs that I saw on channel 26 was on Barbara Scarponi from Portsmouth, New Hampshire. I saw a program on her once before. She is a craftswoman who makes jewelry. It was a fantastic program, beautifully done, and the things she made were beautiful. The area where she lived was beautiful. The program showed her walking by the beach.

When I came home, I was struck by the fact that Frank handled the children so differently than I do. I always tend to contain them. If I'm going to change Katherine's pants, I get everything together that I need in one spot, and I get her, and I put her down and change her, but Frank will say to her, "Go in your room and get a clean diaper," or "Go in your room and get a sweater," or "Go in your room and get a dry shirt," and she goes off, and she might come back or she might not. He's always sending them off. I don't let them do as many things like that because I think it makes such a fantastic mess. He's never afraid of messes, and he's never afraid they're going to fall down or hurt themselves or cut themselves. He'll tell them to go out to the kitchen and get such-and-such. All I think of is that there are knives in the kitchen. They've never had any accidents with Frank. They have all their accidents with me. I'm always the one who is on the edge of my chair, biting my nails, because I'm afraid that they are going to cut themselves, get burnt, fall down, or have some kind of an accident. This tends to make me want to contain them in one spot, get them in one room, while Frank has them running from one end of the house to the other, doing whatever it is they're doing. That's the main difference in the way that we handle them.

When I came home, I was also struck by how differently Thomas and Katherine Louise relate to their toys, to people, to play, and to their environment. Thomas has an amazing fantasy life. He plays with his toys by the hour in a very involved play, and he watches television too. Katherine Louise is only interested in what I'm doing. She's not interested in anything to play with that's just play, like blocks. She was interested in her doll for a while until the new baby came, but she would much rather take out a mop or take silverware out and put it in the dishwasher and take it out again. She's much more interested in manipulating things in the house. Thomas hardly ever touches anything in the house, but Katherine Louise knows where everything is, and wherever it is, she manages to get it. She knows what everything is called and where it goes. She walks around doing little inventories. "Oh, that's Daddy's shirt. Oh, that's Thomas's pajamas." Thomas doesn't seem that aware of the environment in the house. He never starts to play with things like dishes. Katherine Louise tries to make the bed. She tries to dry mop the floor. She likes to put away laundry. She's always playing in the sink. When the two children play at the sink, Thomas does bubbles, she tries to wash dishes. She tries to do things that relate to what I'm doing, whereas the things that he does are pure fantasy play. They are not household tasks watered down to his level.

Those two things struck me. Frank handles the children so differently; I impose many more limits of place on them than Frank does. At the same time, when they're around Frank, they're much more frantic, running back and forth, much more keyed up and excited. He's constantly generating this fantastic excitement as he goes from one spot to another, and they're after him. I'm much more inclined to tell them where we're going or what we're going to do or to do things where they will play quietly while I work things around what they're doing.

Besides Katherine and Thomas and their development and how they react to the new baby, one of the things that's very interesting to me in this new period is comparing notes with my experience after Thomas was born or after Katherine was born, and although after each one was born I tried to at least keep notes, I didn't have my writing going as I do now, and that makes a difference. It is very interesting to compare notes.

I still have some of the same feelings that I had after Thomas was born. Occasionally, I'll recognize that these are the feelings that absolutely frightened me to death after Thomas was born, and I can see it now in a different setting and with a different perspective, and in most cases, it's a feeling that's pint-sized by comparison. Two weeks after I came home from the hospital, I had a checkup with Dr. Kuhn, and Frank's parents watched the children. We went down there and came back, and then Frank's parents left. It was my first time out. It was a thoroughly exhausting experience. We went into Yes, and we went into Canal Mart to look at furniture. I felt as though I could hardly make it back to the car. I was so exhausted. Frank and I were sitting at the table, eating. Frank said to me, "Do you think we should make candles? We could make candles." All of a sudden, I had a really strange feeling. I wanted to say to him, "Are you crazy? How can we make candles? We've got three children under three years of age. We have a newborn. We have so much to do, and you want to spend more time working downstairs? You want to spend more time at your office? You don't even have the dryer hooked up so I can dry the laundry. How can you say, 'Can we make candles?'"

It seems so often that Frank will say to me, "Why don't we make wine?" It seems to me such a big undertaking. It seems to be unbelievable that he'd even suggest it, but that was an instance where it was just getting dark out and I felt so tired and was wondering how many times the baby would get me up that night. Will I be able to make the feeding? Will I be able to get through them? I had the feeling that I'm in the hands of a madman. It is a feeling of generation gone wild. Then, all of a sudden, I catch myself, and I see this pushed further and further. I don't exactly understand this feeling inside me, but I've had it several times when Frank's been talking about why we didn't do this or why we didn't do that. What he's suggesting conjures up to me a picture of us living in an abandoned automobile somewhere, out of touch with reality, like two recluses. A primitive feeling comes over me. I finally told myself, "If he wants to do something like that, there isn't any reason I have to go with him." He probably never would, but whatever it is he's talking about seems to me that this is what he is suggesting, and it used to scare me until I finally decided that I don't have to follow every suggestion he makes. If he decided he wanted to do something like that, I don't necessarily have to do it. I can do whatever I want to. Once I reminded myself of that, it didn't bother me. All of that started me thinking again about the feelings that I had after Thomas was born and why it was the kind of experience that it was. I think that Frank was projecting on to me images of authority, that he was responding to me in the way a small boy responds to his mother. Instead of us having some system for dealing with laundry or shopping, I would have to ask him each time, and each time, he'd feel irritated that I was pressing him. It was like the mother forcing the boy to do something he didn't want to do. It was a horrible hassle over simple things. Having these images, I was afraid I was acting out the role of a stern authority figure. Maybe, I was acting these out because he was projecting them on to me. I do have that potential in myself, and I have been that way at times, and I think it's the side of myself that I like the least. In fact, I hate that side of myself. I think that at that time, I was much closer to my own feelings of hate and hostility and all the qualities that I have that make me less than lovable and all the qualities that I usually suppress. Hate is an aid in recovery. I think that during this recovery time, I am more vulnerable to my own feelings of hate. What happens afterward is that I feel guilty about having these feelings, and I feel I am not worthy of my husband, not worthy of my baby, and not worthy of my other children. I guess that's what can provoke the "blues," the baby blues.

I was really struck by the fact that after the baby was born, I felt as though I had lost all my insides. Frank says that in any change in reality, if you have an operation and have your gall bladder or your kidney removed, you have feelings of loss afterward because you have to adjust to a new physical reality. After the baby was born, I felt like an elevator shaft that had lost its elevator. I felt like an empty husk; I had an empty center. It has something to do with the sex drive being gone because all one's energies, after the baby is born, is directed toward survival of the child and oneself. One doesn't have any center, any dreaminess, or anything that would take one's mind off the task at hand. I feel that I can't get into anything or get involved in anything because I have to keep dealing with surface things all the time.

One of the things regarding this feeling of hate is that I always experience a tremendous annoyance with Frank because I'm always clearing off surfaces. It's the thing that requires to be done more often in this house than anything else. I clear off the kitchen table, the top of the hutch, the top of the bookcase, and the red desk. All the furniture has stuff on it, and I'm forever clearing it off. It's a permanent mental image, and then Frank comes in, and with the stuff in his pockets, the mail he's got, and other things he's brought home, within five minutes after he's home, every surface is covered with stuff. This is a battle that goes on. I fight it out with myself. I wonder why I'm always this way with surfaces. All surfaces of this house and all the counters are the same height. They're about waist high, like the kitchen table, and it's as though I want a taut surface. It's a symbol of my control. I want a taut surface although everything underneath can be junk or stuff stuck there that is similar to the unconscious, like a big wastebasket. As long as the surface is clear, it represents some kind of control.

On Saturday, I called Anna, and I probably talked longer than I should have, but I so much enjoyed talking to her. One of the things she said was that she had been reading the Ulanov book. She said the second part of it is beautiful, where Ulanov explains why there is tremendous emphasis on a woman giving birth to a son. Aside from this being a patriarchal society, she wondered why there always was such emphasis on a woman giving birth to a son. Anna said that Ulanov said that it's similar to a religious experience and that marriage, in a way, is too because it is a way of experiencing the other—and that's why sexuality and spirituality are so close together for women, because both of them are a way of experiencing the "Other," with a capital O—and that the same was true in the birth of a son, for instance, because it came out of you, and it was part of you, and yet it is an "Other." I was reminded of how much I felt this way when Katherine Louise was born. Somehow, to me, she seemed like an object, and Thomas seemed like a subject, and this is how I would characterize it. It did seem different to me that one was a boy and one was a girl.

Yesterday, there was a letter from Emily, and she sent a clipping of an article on feminizing the world by Yoko Ono. There was an interesting quote by James Baldwin in that article saying that after a man performs all day at the office, he can't come home and perform all night with the children, and she commented on the use of the word "performance" and how strange it is that you see this as a performance. As long as men see this as a performance, they certainly aren't going to care to do it. I was thinking about that this morning. Frank had mentioned it, and I was thinking about it because one of the reasons it is so hard for me to care for Thomas and Katherine was that it was like a performance for me; it is like being on the job, like being on duty or on call. It was similar to being on sentry duty. You think that some time, there will come an hour in the day when you're finished, and you can go off duty and do your own thing. The job of motherhood is so overwhelming and demanding that after a while, you have to intrude on your performance. Your personality has to intrude on your performance. Then, at that point, it becomes no longer a performance. Your kids just live with you the way you are. You begin to intrude because otherwise, this little person in you will die, and it would never have a chance to get out. So after a while, it comes out while the kids are there. You are your real self.

Thursday, March 9, 1972

This is coming to the end of my pregnancy with Jennifer. I'm about ready to start a new tape, and I think the new one will be called *Postpartum Papers*. Frank suggested it half-jokingly. For want of anything better, I'm using it as a tribute to his imagination. That's what it will be called.

It's sad for me to close off the pregnancy period. When I was pregnant with Thomas, I was asked, "What does one feel besides the obvious signs and symptoms of pregnancy?" I would say that one of the most blissful and euphoric experiences of my life has been being pregnant. I feel younger. Maybe, it has something to do with my age. Maybe, I wouldn't feel younger if I were twenty-two. I also have a feeling that everything is all right with the world. It's like stepping out on a beautiful day in your favorite season—maybe, it's autumn—and there's a haze in the air or a crackly feeling about everything, or if it's spring, there is a fragrance in the air. I step into a beautiful garden. Things don't bother me so much when I'm pregnant. That's why I described it as feeling as if all is right with the world. Everything is okay.

Now, I'm much more hostile and aggressive. I accept fate less easily when I'm not pregnant, and I rail against it, and I fight it. When I'm pregnant, I ride the waves, the waves of life; I'm carried along and happy to be carried along. While I am pregnant, I feel less in touch with my unconscious and less in touch with the negative side of my own personality, much less in touch with the nightmare side, the bad dream side, the scary side. Everything is an immensely happy dream, beautiful.

I have much more energy when I am pregnant for certain things, not so much for chores. The chores didn't bother me, but I seemed to have more energy for things I really wanted to do and think about, like sorting through papers or notebooks or writing letters to friends. There seemed to be more energy for things that gave me pleasure and less concern about the chores. Everything was in the service of my very inner being, and it was an immensely inward kind of experience, very emotionally satisfying.

I also noticed this time that my personality became totally integrated. Things were knit together at a much deeper level in my psyche than ever before, and I would say that has been the biggest thing in this pregnancy. I certainly noticed it less in my other two pregnancies. Whatever I happened to be thinking about, my unconscious came up with better solutions. Things opened up to me; doors I had been knocking on for a very long time suddenly swung open. It has to do with things that I want to write about, but I suddenly found everything integrated into one whole. All the lines I had been following suddenly began to converge. I had the feeling that all my capabilities were being used. There won't be anything that's innate. Everything is going to be developed, brought forth, represented, embodied, and manifested. I feel more whole and more complete than ever.